Start losing that unnecessary flab around your abs today, with **"Lose Your Stomach Forever"** <u>**The Donnacize Way**</u>. Donna gives you the tools to never worry about belly fat again. Her approach is simple, yet effective as she instructs you in a way that is doable and sensible. Tighten your stomach muscles at work, in the supermarket or while walking your dog.

Problems exercising on the floor. Don't worry, you can exercise your stomach muscles while standing or sitting, no fitness attire required. An easy read that actually works. Donna's instructions are reinforced with step by step photography that catches each move from beginning to end. Don't take short lived, unrealistic actions like starving yourself, participating in fad diets or engaging in improper or unhealthy exercise routines. **"Lose Your Stomach Forever"** <u>**The Donnacize Way**</u> gives you the tools for a lifetime. So what are you waiting for? Lose Your Stomach Today! The Donnacize Way.

Lose Your Stomach Forever

*The Donnacize **Way**(TM)*

Over 100 Pictures

Over 40 Stomach Exercises
In order to Lose Your Stomach You

MUST *know these three building blocks*

Donna Lynn

International Instructor, Producer & Host of Morning Exercise Program, Owner & Founder of Donnacize Aerobics Inc.

Bloomington, IN Milton Keynes, UK

authorHOUSE™

AuthorHouse™
1663 Liberty Drive, Suite 200
Bloomington, IN 47403
www.authorhouse.com
Phone: 1-800-839-8640

AuthorHouse™ UK Ltd.
500 Avebury Boulevard
Central Milton Keynes, MK9 2BE
www.authorhouse.co.uk
Phone: 08001974150

First published by AuthorHouse 2/07/2006

ISBN: 1-4259-0553-6 (sc)

Printed in the United States of America
Bloomington, Indiana

This book is printed on acid-free paper.

Photographer- Jeffrey Butler
Hair- Caron Cuffie
Illustrator- Eric Cuffie
Designer- Michelle Curbeam
Copy Editor- York Eggleston IV

I truly believe that by utilizing this book, you can change your life forever.   But, as we are all at different levels of physical fitness, please be sure to consult your physician prior to starting any exercise program.

Table of Contents

Acknowledgements

I am extremely thankful for my mother who was quiet, cute and possessed the most beautiful spirit. Thank you for my happy childhood and my life as it is today. I still have not met anyone who can in the same moment possess your strength and calmness.

To my dad who taught discipline and a strong faith belief system. Thanks for the life lessons I continue to use on a daily basis. Although you both have passed, you still live within me in so many ways.

To my loving and handsome son Tyrell. Thank you for helping to make Donnacize what it is today. Many people would love to have a son who is articulate, smart, and well mannered. You have been a blessing since day one.

Without my family's support I would not have been able to fully live my dreams. So, thank you Margie for all the hours you put in at Donnacize Aerobic Studio. I could not have done it without you. Thank you Gail, for your support, enthusiasm and encouraging words. Winston, for teaching my line dance classes and Larry, Kelvin, Anthony and Paulette for being wonderful siblings. To my beautiful and talented niece Pat, thank you for instructing my classes. I can't wait to see where your talents will take you.

To all of my Aunts, Uncles, Cousins, nieces, nephews and in-laws, especially Cousin Cliff (junior) I love you like a brother. I don't see you as often as I would like, but I feel blessed to be a part of such a strong family.

I want to thank my brother-in-law, Eric Cuffie, for all of the artwork he's created for me over the years, including the wonderful drawings in this book.

Special thanks to Mr. York Eggelston IV. I have yet to meet a man as passionate, intelligent and articulate as you are. You helped "shape" this book and I am forever grateful and thankful for your opinion, time and energy.

Michelle Curbeam, thank you for stepping up to the plate as an instructor and designer. You are extremely talented and I wish you the best as you pursue your dreams. Thank you Jeffrey Butler of Jazzy Photos, for taking the photographs for this book and for always being a great friend. Your patience and professionalism goes above and beyond the call of duty. Joann Elkeldo, thank you again and again. You have always believed in my projects and included me in yours, my complete gratitude to you. Mr. Donald Hutchins and the Sojourner-Douglass family, thanks for your support and encouragement.

To my friends Jacqueline Trader, Pat Allen and Donna Chiarella, thank you for always being there and taking time to listen to my personal and business issues.

There have been so many people who have helped "form" my career. To all the patrons of Donnacize Aerobics Studio, you could have taken your business elsewhere, but you decided to build with me. Thank you all! If it had not been for you, there would have been no studio. You were all so amazing and I am thankful and grateful for your presence.

To my clients who are currently exercising and supporting me, Thank you! Thank you! And thank you again! I am so grateful for your spirits, your time, and your energy. You are all so WONDERFUL!

I know I have left many family members, friends and associates out who have also been a part of my life in a big way. Please accept my apology and this thank you is for you. THANK YOU!!!!!!!!!!!!!!

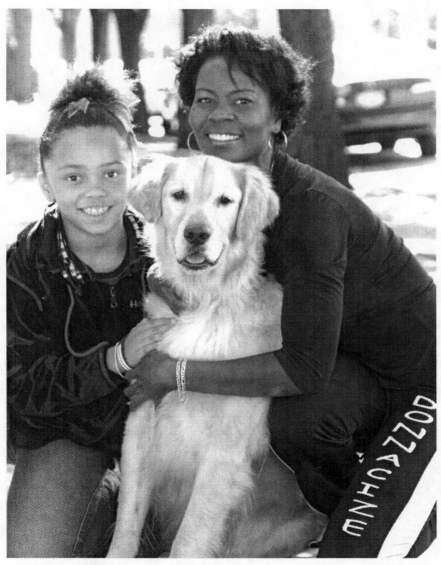

My Goddaughter Toni and My Dog Baxter after a Saturday Morning Walk.

I decided to write this book after encountering thousands of men and women, both internationally and nationally, who when asked what they are physically trying to accomplish stated, *"I just want to lose my stomach."* You too may share similar concerns. These men and women, whose ages, races, nationalities and yes, sizes were as diverse as the colors in a rainbow, all found themselves in the same predicament. This book will serve as a guide to help rid yourself of unnecessary pounds and that unwanted pouch.

Hi, my name is Donna Lynn and I'm excited to become a part of your healthy lifestyle. Working out is a part of my job. If I don't look the part, my clients will go to someone else who does. That's pretty strong motivation to stay physically fit. I stay in shape, particularly in the abdominal region, by paying attention to three basic building blocks for a healthy lifestyle the "Donnacize™ Way": **diet, exercise routine,** and **posture**. My goal is to get these three parts of your life working for you just as I have done for my clients and myself. So, even if your goal is to get rid of your stomach, you must start with your diet. For example, a high protein diet makes me full longer and keeps my stomach flat, whereas eating too many carbohydrates makes me feel bloated. As you become stronger, healthier and more aware of your body, you too will learn what foods make you feel full, bloated or light.

In addition, just like you, my life does not afford me the luxury of doing crunches all day, and my life is just as hectic and unpredictable as yours. I work, have a son, attend graduate school, I'm on the staff at a college where I teach over 100 students, AND I'm not a kid anymore. As a fitness professional for over 15 years, I've heard it all from, "I don't have the time to exercise", to "If I exercise too often I'll mess up my hair." Believe me, it's not about the time and it's not about the hair. Changing from an unhealthy lifestyle to a healthy one is about re-prioritizing how you eat, think and feel.

If you want to see your abdominal muscles, you have to get rid of what's hiding them. To do this you must exercise and accomplish two simple dietary goals:

* Eat enough to preserve muscle
* Don't eat so much that you put on fat

This may not seem easy, but it's very doable, which is why we talk about Burning the Fat, Mini Meals, the importance of Fruit and Vegetables, Protein, and much more in Chapters III and VIII.

A contract to yourself is also enclosed in Chapter II for the days extra motivation is needed (and believe me, there will be those days). We move to the book's highlight and learn how to properly exercise the rectus abdominal area, the internal and external oblique muscles, and the lower stomach muscles in Section II. Chapters VII, III and IX reveal the importance of bringing it all together with lower back exercises and the importance of posture. Many people fail to realize that in order to achieve a wispy waistline the lower back muscles must also be toned. The lower back muscles are the opposing muscle group of the abdominal area. When one is strengthened alone, the other becomes weaker, so please exercise both. Posture is another forgotten force of a fitness regimen. If you do not carry your body weight properly you are exercising in vain, whether you move aerobically seven days a week or not, you will fail to see the results you've worked so hard for.

Chapter VIII stress the importance of drinking water and will immediately motivate you to drink an extra glass or two per day. The last section, but definitely not the least, consist of three empowering chapters, "You Are Not Alone", "Feeling Good About You" and "Questions I'm Most Often Asked". These chapters were created as a reminder that others have gone through and will continue to go through the same trials you're experiencing, and just like them you can and will succeed. So be inspired and know that at the end of the day you too can change your body and improve the quality of your life.

This book is designed to be doable and fun. The exercises can be done at work or in the privacy of your home. The book is purposefully sized to fit easily into your purse or handbag, and should serve as your health reference and motivational assistant. To make this a rewarding, and learning experience, please take a moment to ask yourself a few questions:

1. **What are my short term goals?** Ex. In three months I will finally zip up the jeans I haven't worn in over three years.

2. **What are my long term goals:** Ex. I will lose 30 pounds by the end of the year.

3. **How can I incorporate healthy living into my lifestyle.** Ex. Every Monday, Wednesday and Friday I will exercise at 6:30 am.

4. **What small changes can I make in pursuit of a healthier diet?** Ex. My last meal will be eaten four hours before bedtime.

These goals will help focus you. You see, until fitness becomes a part of your lifestyle, any distraction or excuse is a reason not to move. These distractions come in a variety of forms and can be as simple as a phone call, a television program you've been wanting to watch or even a sale at the mall. Once you decide what your goals are, write them down on your calendar or post them on your mirror. These will serve as reminders to help you stay focused. Also realize that losing pounds and inches will require self-discipline, hard work and sacrifice. So if you're ready to commit, I will become your training partner in the privacy of your home. Everything that we accomplish first starts with a thought and desire which you obviously must have. So if you're ready, let's, **"Lose Your Stomach Forever, the Donnacize Way.**

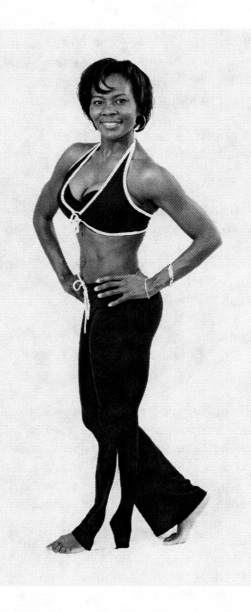

Section I:

The Donnacize Way

Chapter I
5 Principles Of
The Donnacize Way

The Donnacize Way is a philosophy that is embodied in the writings, teachings and classes of Donnacize, Inc., all aimed at promoting and maintaining a well balanced and rewarding lifestyle. At the core of its philosophy, five basic principles guide both the instructors and students of the Donnacize Way:

* You Must Commit To A Healthy Lifestyle For You And Only You

Take responsibility for your health and commit to a healthier lifestyle. If you put in the work, the results will come. You must do this for YOU!

* Three Regimental Building Blocks Must Become A Part Of Your Life

1. **Diet-** A healthy diet is not about starving or depriving yourself. A healthy diet is about making good food choices that will enhance the way you look and feel.

2. **Exercise-** You must move aerobically 20-30 minutes 3-4 times per week. Unlike objects that wear over time, the body becomes stronger and healthier when it's strengthened and taken out of its comfort zone.

3. **Posture-** This is the major building block that make everything work. Good posture is the foundation of a strong healthy body. When you understand the importance of good posture, then you begin to see how the body works and functions properly. This allows you to exercise more intelligently.

These 3 Building Blocks done in harmony are the foundation to a successful and healthy lifestyle.

* An Exercise Regimen Should be Fun And Uncomplicated

If you're going to move aerobically and sweat, you should have fun. Donna Lynn and her staff understand the importance of our clients being motivated to stick with a program that's enjoyed. This is why our fitness classes are full of energy and fun. They are challenging enough to take you to a variety of levels, yet simple enough to perform at home.

* Variety In Exercise Really Is The Spice Of Fitness

We are all multi-faceted and multi-talented. So it makes sense that an exercise program has a variety of elements to suit our mood, fitness level and personality. The Donnacize way is a philosophy that is embodied in the writings, teachings and classes comprised of a long, exciting and challenging list of classes that range from, but are not limited to The Donnacize Groove, Get Funky and Move, Pilates, Muscle Conditioning and Lo-Impact Aerobics.

* Fitness Must Be Consistent To Have A Lasting Impact

Consistency is the key. In order to see change you must change your previous schedule and make exercising a priority. Choose to move aerobically 3-4 times per week without fail. DON'T MAKE EXCUSES. A half hearted exercise schedule, gives you half hearted results. In order for fitness to have a lasting impact you must consistently move as a lifestyle.

These principles were created to guide you through a fitness and lifestyle program. The benefits and highlights of the principles is that if only one is put into action major changes are still seen. Choose one philosophy and commit to it without fail. And when one becomes a natural part of your daily routine add another. The fit can enjoy a lifestyle that the unfit cannot. Choose to be fit!

Chapter 2:
"Donnacize Lose Your Stomach Forever" Contract

This Donnacize contract is your commitment to yourself and no one else. It will help focus and motivate you on the days when you need reinforcement and really just don't want to move, let alone do stomach exercises. Commitment just means keeping your promises to yourself. If you say you are going to eat meat twice a week or exercise four times per week, then you should do exactly that. The only diet that it takes to lose weight is the one that you stick to. The only exercise program it takes to get your heart rate and fitness to a good level, is the one you stick to. *Either you are committed or you're not.* Commitment means doing what it takes to get results, no matter what. So when your schedule gets tight, **Don't Quit**, "COMMIT". When your work schedule changes, **Don't Quit**, "COMMIT". Redesign your schedule and continue to move forward.

<u>Do not over extend yourself</u>. Make sure you choose realistic steps to achieving your short and long term goals. State exactly how often you will exercise your cardiovascular system along with the number of stomach exercises you will do per day.

Over the years, the time of day to exercise has worked really well for me. Whether it's early morning, or before bedtime, I become very selfish with my time and it doesn't change for anyone. I also reward myself when I've accomplished a goal. You too should determine a reward for yourself every month just for sticking with your contract. It should be something meaningful to you that would be celebratory of a job well done. This can be anything from a night out dancing, a champagne toast, a new outfit or a healthy dessert you've been meaning to try.

Once you complete your Donnacize Contract, post it where it can be seen daily. Research shows that one of the best ways

als)

Chapter III:
3 Building Blocks that Will Change Your Waistline Forever

The following three Building Blocks are what makes your healthy lifestyle work together. They are the fundamental tools needed to change your waistline forever. It doesn't matter what you are physically trying to accomplish, you cannot skip these fundamentals if you want to see a change. Proper technique, diet and exercise will give you the tools to change your body for a lifetime. Make the building blocks a part of your daily tasks and your fitness level will rise.

Building Block 1: Diet

When talking to men and women about their eating habits, I am amazed by the large number who skip meals. Many of them are of the opinion that skipping meals will increase their weight-loss. This is absolutely not true. In fact it has the opposite effect. Skipping meals slows down the metabolism and allows the body to store more fat. People who purposely skip meals in order to lose weight often find that they are hungrier and resort to binge eating. It's much healthier to eat planned, controlled meals. These types of scheduled meals can put an end to emotional eating.

For a second, let's forget about healthy eating to lose weight. Let's focus on healthy eating for longevity, healthy eating to enjoy an active lifestyle with your family and most importantly healthy eating to feel good about you. You see, many people believe that in order to lose weight you must starve yourself or eat tasteless foods. Again, this is simply not true. In order to lose weight you must exercise and cut back on fried, high calorie foods. Once these foods become a limited part of your diet, you want to replace them with foods that are full of vitamins and minerals. It's essential to get a colorful variety of fruit and vegetables into your diet every day, because colorful fruit and vegetables provide the wide range of vitamins, minerals and fiber your body uses to stay healthy and energetic. Try starting the day with fruit or an 8-ounce glass of 100 percent juice such as orange or grapefruit. A sliced banana or berries on your bran or wheat cereal can also give you a delicious, low-fat, high-fiber head start.

Also, remember that fruit and vegetables are portable and can give you a quick boost of flavor and energy at anytime. Pack an apple or a bag of carrot sticks, raisins, or dried apricots into your glove compartment, purse or briefcase. These fruit and vegetables contain anti-oxidants like beta carotene and vitamins C and E, and they help to maintain a healthy weight, protect against the effects of aging, and reduce the risk of cancer and heart disease. The National Cancer Institute is researching the way these foods protect health. The nutrients are famed for their ability to vanquish free radicals which are harmful molecules that circulate in the body and damage healthy tissue. Read on to find out what's in some of the food you eat:

Bananas - This fruit may help lower blood pressure. The magic ingredient? Potassium. Bananas are also rich in vitamin B6, which research shows to be essential in maintaining a strong immune system.

Barley - This is brimming with beta glucans, a type of soluble fiber that can lower your risk of heart disease by reducing levels of artery-clogging LDL (low-density lipo-proteins). Hull-less, waxy varieties contain the most beta glucans. Look for the term "unpearled" on the box, meaning unprocessed and thus higher in fiber, which helps lower blood pressure.

Beef (lean)- Lean beef may help ward off infections and protect against cellular damage that can lead to cancer. That's because lean beef is an excellent source of niacin, which may prevent cancerous changes, and zinc, an immune-strengthener.

Black beans - These and other beans are full of soluble fiber, which helps lower LDL and reduce blood pressure. It also helps keep blood sugar levels on an even keel, staving off hunger and even reducing the need for insulin among diabetics.

Bran cereal - Choose one high in wheat bran, a great source of cancer-fighting insoluble fiber, which increases stool bulk and speed of elimination. (Scientists think that the faster toxins move through your bowels, the lower your risk of colo-rectal cancer.) Look for a cereal that provides at least 5 grams of fiber per serving.

Broccoli - Broccoli is bursting with cancer-fighting fiber, beta carotene and vitamin C, plus boron, bone-building calcium, chromium, folic acid and potassium.

Brown rice - This contains oryzanol, which can reduce LDL. The high-fiber rice bran found in brown rice may help lower cholesterol. Brown rice also contains copper, magnesium, niacin, thiamine, vitamins B6 and E, which can strengthen the immune system and reduce the risk of heart disease and cataracts, and zinc.

Cabbage - A member of the cruciferous family of cancer-fighting vegetables, its anti-cancer key may be the presence of indoles, one of which may help prevent breast cancer.

Cantaloupe - This is brimming with beta carotene, fiber, folate potassium and vitamins B6 and C. Carotene's anti-cancer effect may protect against oral cancers as well as cancers of the cervix, stomach and uterus.

Carrots - Best for their sky-high beta carotene content. A recent study of 87,000 women found that those who ate five or more servings of carrots a week were 68 percent less likely to suffer a stroke than those eating one or fewer carrots a month.

Figs - Figure on getting fiber, magnesium, potassium and vitamin C from figs. A recent study at Harvard School of Public Health found that only fruit fiber, like that found in figs, is linked to reduced systolic blood pressure (the upper number, which represents pressure during the heart's contractions). All fiber is associated with reduced diastolic blood pressure (the lower number, which represents the pressure when the heart is at rest between contractions).

Fish - The omega-3 fatty acids in fish oils are the fix for lowering blood fats, especially triglycerides. They also help reduce blood pressure and may ease arthritis symptoms. Anchovies, bluefish, herring, lake trout, mackerel, salmon and sardines have the most fatty acids.

Garlic - Research suggests garlic helps protect against heart disease and stroke. It may also lower blood pressure. Garlic also contains allylic sulfides, which may detoxify carcinogens. It also has been linked to lower rates of stomach cancer.

Ginger - This may be a natural diet aid, possibly boosting the rate at which the body burns calories. It's also a natural antioxidant.

Grapes - Grapes are a great source of boron, a mineral that may help ward off osteoporosis.

Kale - Another boon against heart disease, this vegetable is especially rich in beta carotene, calcium, copper, fiber, manganese, potassium and vitamins B6 and C.

Kiwi fruit - Its fuzzy brown exterior hides a bright green interior chock-full of cancer- fighting fiber and vitamin C.

Lentils - A powerhouse of nutrients especially B vitamins, which may help protect against heart attacks. Lentils are also high in fiber, minerals such as iron and immune-boosting copper, manganese and zinc, and protein.

Mango - These luscious fruits are just brimming with beta carotene, copper, and vitamin B6 and C.

Miso - This soybean paste, used to season soups and sauces, contains isoflavones, which may protect against breast cancer.

Nuts - These help your heart. A study at Loma Linda University in California found that adults on a low-fat diet who ate 2 ounces of walnuts five or more times a week lowered their total cholesterol levels by 12 percent. A control group followed the same diet, minus the nuts, showed just a 6 percent drop.

Oats - A good choice for lowering LDL cholesterol. Recent studies suggest eating 3 grams of soluble fiber a day, the amount in a large bowl of 100 percent oat-bran cereal can cut LDL cholesterol by 5 percent in six weeks.

Olive oil - Olive oil is the richest in mono-unsaturated fats, which may lower blood cholesterol. A recent study found that LDL cholesterol can be cut by some 7 percent by substituting olive oil for margarine- more if replacing butter.

Orange juice - This classic source of vitamin C also contains folic acid, which helps prevent birth defects and may protect against cervical cancer.

Pears - A super source of fiber, which, when combined with a low-fat diet, can lessen the risk of developing polyps in the colon, a precursor to cancer. Pears also provide boron, potassium and vitamin C.

Prunes - These are constipation relievers because of their fiber and sorbitol, a natural sugar. They also contains boron and vitamins A and E.

Pumpkin - The fall favorite is very high in carotene, just like its winter squash cousins, butternut and hubbard. All are fiber rich.

Red bell peppers - A better anti-cancer pick than green peppers because they contain extra carotenes. They also supply more potassium and vitamin C.

Skim milk - The best source of bone-building calcium and riboflavin, a b vitamin that helps maintain energy.

Spinach - A powerhouse of antioxidants and nutrients. It's particularly rich in folic acid, which may protect against cervical dysplasia, a condition that precedes cervical cancer.

Strawberries - These berries contain more vitamin c and fiber than most fruits, including oranges. (In fact, all berries are excellent sources of fiber.) Strawberries also contain ellagic acid, a natural cancer fighting chemical.

Sunflower seeds - These are similar to nuts in polyunsaturated fat content, but with much more vitamin E.

Sweet potatoes - These pack twice as much fiber and significantly more beta carotene than white or red potatoes.

Tea - Many studies describe the chemicals in tea that may prevent cancer as well as lower blood cholesterol. Most of the research has been on green tea, but there is some evidence of similar benefits from oolong tea.

Tomatoes - These contain lycopene, which may prevent some cancers. They also supply fiber and potassium, as well as vitamins A and C.

Wheat germ - Top notch for almost any nutrient. Just a 1/4 cup packs 5 grams of fiber, as well as B vitamins, iron, magnesium and zinc. It's also rich in chromium, manganese and vitamin E.

Whole wheat bread - Whole wheat bread contains triple the fiber found in white bread and is richer in magnesium and vitamin B6.

Yogurt - The ultimate health food, yogurt may prevent colds and allergy attacks. It's also a super source of bone-building calcium.

MINI MEALS

Mini meals are a recommended way to eat when trying to lose weight. You are not depriving yourself to the point of hunger and you eat throughout the day without feeling bogged down and tired. Mini meals also help to speed up your body's metabolism (which is the rate at which your body burns calories). By eating small meals every 3 to 4 hours, your body knows it's constantly going to be nourished and therefore burns calories instead of storing most of them.

On a daily basis, we need six nutrients to live:

* Carbohydrates - like potatoes, rice, pastas and bread

Carbohydrates are an excellent energy source that protects the muscles in the body. They are the food group that when overlooked and overloaded turns into fat. That's why monitoring your carbohydrate intake along with exercising is one of the single most important things you can do. Carbohydrates can be divided into two categories: simple carbohydrates and complex carbohydrates. Simple carbohydrates are generally associated with a low-nutrient density and include honey, corn syrup, and refined sugars such as table sugar. Complex carbohydrates are those carbohydrate sources that are nutrient dense, such as whole grains, vegetables, and fruits. They are typically high in essential vitamins and minerals, contain longer chain sugars (polysaccharides) and contain dietary fiber. The USDA recommends that 55-60% of the total number of calories consumed be in the form of carbohydrates.

* Proteins like beans, fish, poultry, plants, egg whites and a variety of meats are used to build new cells, maintain tissues, and synthesize new proteins that make it possible for you to perform basic bodily functions. Protein is found in meat, poultry, fish and dried peas and beans (legumes). It is also present in dairy products. To get the protein your body needs without taking in unnecessary fat and cholesterol, select lean cuts of meat, poultry without skin, and fish. Protein supplies the body with amino acids. Amino acids are absorbed and used primarily to build new and rebuild damaged body proteins such as hair, skin, muscles, cartilage, hemoglobin, enzymes, hormones, and various proteins in the blood. Unused amino acids are stored as body fat. The waste products from fat conversion must be excreted in the urine, requiring additional work for the kidneys. While protein provides the basic building blocks for body tissues, research has not shown that megadoses of protein (amino acids) will increase muscle tissue growth during training or contribute significantly to energy needs.

Fats

Many of us think of fat in terms of body fat, we have too much and we want to get rid of it. This may be true, but eaten in moderation fat has a vital function in our lives. Fat cushions our vital internal organs, insulate our bodies, and stores energy for later use. Our problems arise when we don't burn enough energy to use stored fat, that's why exercising is so important. Fats provide more than twice the energy as the same amount of protein or carbohydrates. They are important in energy production, temperature regulation and distribution of vitamins A, D, E and K.

* There are 2 different groups of fat:

Saturated fats are usually found in meat and dairy products and are solid at room temperature. The vegetable oil from palm kernel, coconut, palm, and cocoa oils also contain large proportions of saturated fat. Too many saturated fats can clog your arteries and increase your chances of heart disease, so please eat them sparingly.

Unsaturated fats are usually liquid at room temperature and are generally associated with plant sources and includes fats like olive oil, canola oil and natural peanut butter. Fish and chicken also contain unsaturated fats. It is heart wise to cook with mono or polyunsaturated fats versus saturated fats.

* Minerals - You get these from your fruit and vegetables. Minerals are elements that originate in the Earth and cannot be made by living systems. Plants obtain minerals from the soil, and most of the minerals in our diets come directly from plants or indirectly from animal sources. Minerals are inorganic chemical elements that must be present for the maintenance of health. They are important for body structures and for controlling body processes, but do not supply calories. Except for iron, minerals are not used up in the body, but are excreted after carrying out his or her respective functions. This is why mineral losses must be replaced regularly. Four of the minerals that are found in the largest quantities are calcium, iron, magnesium, and potassium.

* Water - Water is the single most important nutrient you take in every day. It makes up more than one-half your body weight. It's fat-free, cholesterol free, low in sodium and completely without calories. Proper hydration is essential for energy production because water is the medium in which all metabolic reactions take place. Fluids regulate body temperature and carry nutrients to cells, aid in digestion and excretion of waste products, and are necessary for all chemical reactions within the body. Most adults need at least 8-10 (8 ounce) glasses of water per day. Dark gold urine may indicate a water deficiency assuming no influence from medications or nutrient supplements. Athletes and people living in hot climates require considerably more. Water is so important that, without it, your body just can't work.

Nonessential Nutrients

Fiber

Dietary fiber is a nonessential nutrient that is worth taking a moment to talk about. Dietary fiber aids in proper digestion and consists of the indigestible components of plants. The easiest way to increase fiber content in the diet is to increase consumption of unrefined carbohydrates such as whole-grain breads, cereals, root vegetables, yams, potatoes, and fruits. Humans do not possess the necessary enzymes to digest fiber; instead, they pass through the digestive system in the same form as they were ingested rendering fiber unusable as energy. It is recommended that people consume 20-35 grams of fiber per day to help prevent cancers of the digestive system, hemorrhoids, constipation, and diverticular diseases.

Building Block 2: Exercise - BURNING FAT

MADE SIMPLE AND EASY

The good news about exercise is that it doesn't take long workouts at a fitness club to get in shape. You can work out intensely and burn belly fat without leaving the privacy of your home. For the inactive person, this is a great way to get in shape in a comfortable, non-intimidating environment. For the person who's already active, you may want to increase the duration or intensity of exercise by incorporating strength training into your routine. This section give options on how to burn fat and keep it off. The exercises below are chosen for there simplicity, and can be done in or outdoors:

* If you're a beginner, start by walking 10 minutes to warm up. Walk fast for 5-10 minutes, then do 10-15 squats, repeat the walking and squat sequence at least 3 more times. After that, walk for 5-10 minutes to cool down.

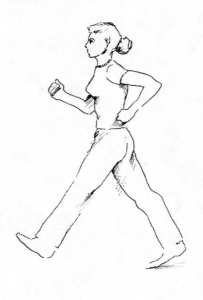

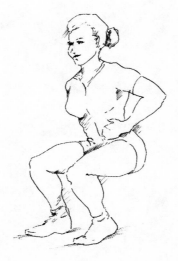

* Intermediate- When the beginner's workout start to feel less challenging, walk fast for 10 minutes to warm up. Jog for 10-15 minutes, then do 10 knee lifts and 10 squats,   Repeat the sequence at least 3 times or more. Walk to cool down.

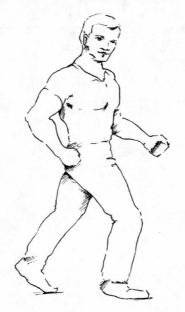

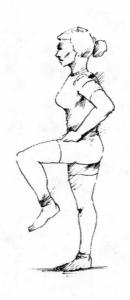

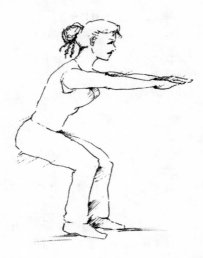

* Advanced - Jog for 10-15 minutes to warm up. Walk fast for 5-10 minutes, jog again for 15 minutes, walk fast for 5 minutes, repeat this sequence at least 3 times, end with 20 knee lifts and 20 squats, complete 2 sets

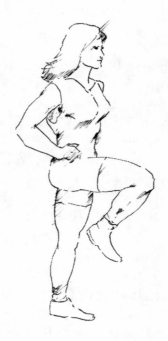

* Speed walk to run local errands, after work or even during lunch breaks.

* Put on your favorite cd and vacuum to a faster beat.

* While watching television, sit on the floor and stretch, do leg lifts or stomach exercises.

* Ride a stationary or mobile bicycle.

* Gather the kids and jog through the neighborhood.

* While at work if you're going up less than three flights in a building ALWAYS use the stairs instead of the elevator.

* Tired of walking the pavements? Try hitting the trails with your family or friends and plan a hiking trip.

* Take an aerobics class at your local recreation center. Some community churches also offer free or low priced exercise classes.

* While you're at home, turn off the television and dance to music with your family for at least thirty minutes. This family activity is so much fun that you may find yourself dancing much longer than planned.

These simple activities can make a world of difference when decreasing your body fat. If you are reading this book, there is a good chance that you are living an inactive lifestyle. **Remember, the fit can enjoy a lifestyle that the unfit cannot, BE FIT!**

Building Block 3: POSTURE
Your stomach can never be as flat as possible without good posture. Good posture will automatically give you

a stomach that appears flatter and have you looking taller, trimmer, and fitter.

As a child I'm pretty sure we've heard those admonishing words more than once from our mothers and teachers, "Sit up straight ", and "Don't Slouch". Our immediate response was to lift our upper bodies higher, still not knowing if our posture was good or not, just hoping that it was better. Good posture basically refers to the body's alignment and positioning with respect to the force of gravity. It is the position in which you hold your body upright against gravity while standing, sitting or lying down.

Half the battle of losing stomach fat is gaining good posture. Poor postural habits can increase a waistline by 2-3 inches even if you exercise on a daily basis. Why? Because even the slightest slouch brings weight forward and that weight goes straight to the belly. In order to attain good posture and alleviate those dreadful inches, follow the steps for good posture and review illustration number one.

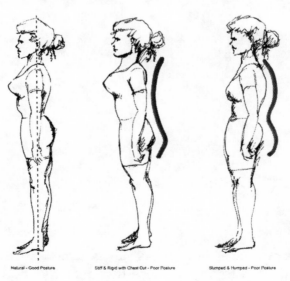

Natural - Good Posture   Stiff & Rigid with Chest Out - Poor Posture   Slumped & Humped - Poor Posture

GOOD POSTURE
Head up,
Chin level with floor,
Chest up
Shoulders relaxed,
Lower abdomen flat

CENTER LINE
Extends from center of head,
through neck, shoulder, hips,
knees and arches of feet

BODY WEIGHT
Body weight is balanced along
the center line and supported
by the weight-bearing arches
of the feet

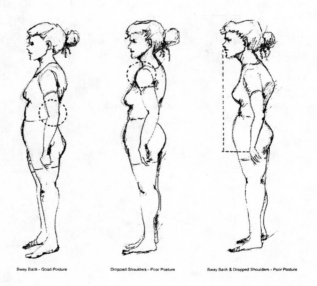

Sway Back - Good Posture   Dropped Shoulders - Poor Posture   Sway Back & Dropped Shoulders - Poor Posture

Good posture on a daily basis, takes time and effort. Poor posture can lead to one of these five defective body postures that are seen way too often. They can lead to a protruding stomach, lower and upper back pain and stiff joints.   Take this time to evaluate your own posture and begin to work on it daily.

So, remember as you eat a healthy diet and include regular exercise and toning to your schedule, practice good posture. This will bring you closer to a flat stomach while at work, home, sitting, standing or walking.   Practicing good posture will keep those unnecessary inches away from your mid-section and you will enjoy a taller, leaner and healthier body.

Section II:

Exercises to Trim That Waistline

Chapter 4:
Rectus Abdominal
Exercises

The abdominal area is really one long segmented muscle which includes four basic areas. These four muscle groups combine to completely cover the internal organs. The abdominal muscles are located between the ribs and the pelvis on the front of the body. They support the trunk, allow movement, and hold organs in place by regulating internal abdominal pressure. The abdominal group is one of the most exercised muscle groups. Usually a few sets of many repetitions are utilized to enhance the core's endurance, and assist the muscles with one of their main functions within the body. Stomach muscles are used as stabilizers, which facilitate many other movements our body perform. Because of this, they require much endurance in order to support the spine, enhance lower back functioning, and accommodate our many activities. Although endurance is important, strengthening these muscles is equally important. You will know what part of the abdominal you're working as you read the chapter heading and the exercise instructions.

The four main abdominal muscles are:

*Transversus abdominus** - the deepest muscle layer. Its main roles are to stabilize the trunk and maintain internal abdominal pressure.

*Rectus abdominus** - slung between the ribs and the pubic bone at the front of the pelvis. This muscle has the characteristic bumps or bulges, when contracting, that are commonly called "the six pack". The main function of the rectus abdominus is to move the body between the ribcage and the pelvis.

*External oblique muscles- these flank the rectus abdominus. The external oblique muscles allow the trunk to twist, but to the opposite side of whichever external oblique is contracting. For example, the right external oblique contracts to turn the body to the left.

> ***Internal oblique muscles**- these flank the rectus abdominus, and are located just inside the hip bones. They operate in the opposite way to the external oblique muscles. For example, twisting the trunk to the left requires the left hand side internal oblique and the right hand side external oblique to contract together.

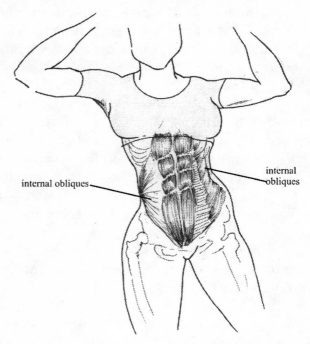

internal obliques

internal obliques

Standing stomach exercises are provided for those with back problems or who are uncomfortable lying on the floor. Also included are moderations for a variety of the exercises when the original movement appears too difficult. Please do not feel pressured to move to the advanced exercises before first feeling comfortable with the basic movement. You should take time to read the instructions carefully and try to complete at least 2 sets of 10, adding on as you become stronger.   This is done to insure that your form is correct. Also remember that the best breathing technique is to exhale upon exertion. Breathing out as you lift your shoulders decreases internal air pressure, allowing you to fully involve the transverse abdominal (the muscle responsible for pulling the tummy in and up). So remember, while at work, sitting, standing or at home, you too can **"Lose Your Stomach Forever, *The Donnacize Way*."**

Breathing Exercise/ Sitting Position

In a comfortable sitting position, lift through the abdominal area, shoulders are down, chest is out. This exercise is the perfect first step to beginning your stomach exercises. You're oxygenating every cell, controlling every muscle, becoming aware of your body and feeling present.

A. Sitting on the floor, knees are bent with your hands under thighs, shoulders are down, your chest is out, your back is flat and your stomach is tight

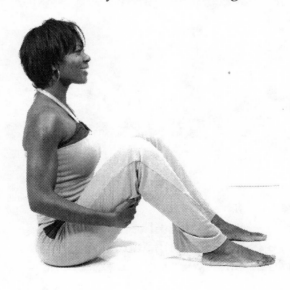

B. Breathe, inhale thru the nose and exhale
thru the mouth. Keep hands under your
thighs and hold position.
Try to repeat 5 times

The next four exercises are core stabilization exercises. They are those activities that don't necessarily target a specific group of muscles, but rather focus on utilizing all of the trunk musculature (anterior and posterior) to stabilize the spine with or without movement.

Pelvic Stability (Leg Slides)

Your pelvic area should sink into your mat. Keep your movement fluent and do not jerk.
A. Lie on your back,
your lower

back should be pressed into the floor
(Arms at your side
palms flat on the floor, fingertips
toward your feet. Legs are straight.

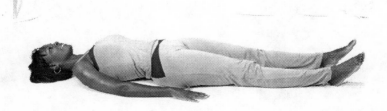

B. Slide your right leg in until your knee
is bent. Keep your pelvic still and palms
flat on the floor. Slide your right leg back out

Repeat on your left leg, (Try not to push
your leg into the floor too much while keeping
pelvic still)

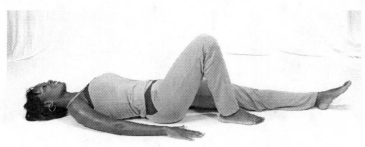

Stabilizing Scapula

You're creating a mood and "an energy." This exercise is going to help you feel the stabilityof your torso. Keep chest and shoulders stable. The move is coming from the abdominal area. Your back should sink into the floor. Keep your movement fluent (Do not jerk). You should feel this stretch across the chest and arms.

A. Lie on your back knees are bent,
arms open shoulder level, (Make sure your back
is flat on the floor)

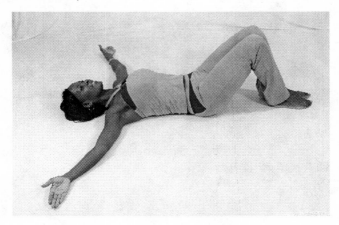

29

B. Inhale as you bring your
arms together reaching towards the
ceiling, palms facing each other, arms
shoulder width apart

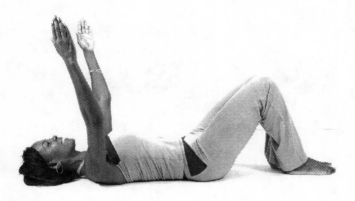

C. Exhale and open your arms for 4 counts, feel the
stretch across the chest and the arms (keep
arms half an inch above the ground)

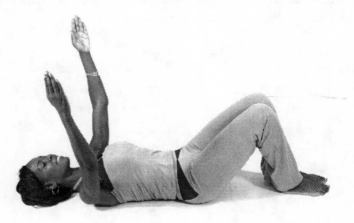

Repeat at least 10 times

Core Stabilization Full Body Plank

A. Keep the neck aligned with the rest of the spine
B. Engage the abdominal area throughout the exercise to stabilize the pelvis and spine

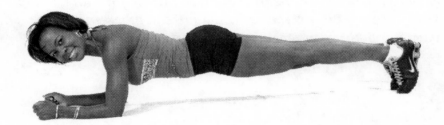

(Full Body Plank)

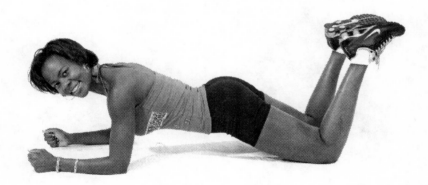

(Bent Knee Plank)

Proper Body Technique for Abdominal Exercises

* Keep the neck in line with the rest of the spine and a space between the chin and chest
* Keep abdominal muscles tightly contracted throughout the exercise to prevent the lower back from arching off the mat and the rib cage popping out

* The main concern is not to pull on the neck in trying to increase range of motion
* Keep spine neutral and legs and gluteal relaxed

Our Stomach section begins with a basic crunch. The only thing needed is your body and your will. The movement is easy to do and puts absolutely no strain on your lower back. When doing the exercises, always remember that form is very important, so read the instructions carefully.

The Basic Stomach Crunch #1

A. Lie on your back with your knees bent
and feet flat on the floor. Press your
lower back firmly into the floor
Rest your head into your hands. Keep your chin lifted and
    your neck and shoulders relaxed

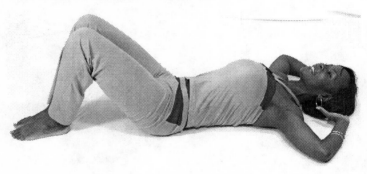

B. Exhale as you lift your shoulders off the floor
for 1 count and inhale as you go back for 1 count

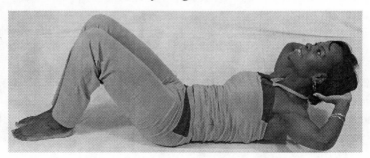

Try to complete 20-30 times adding on as you become stronger

Cradle Crunch #2

A. Lie on your back with your knees bent. Place your fingers behind your head, with your elbows open to the sides

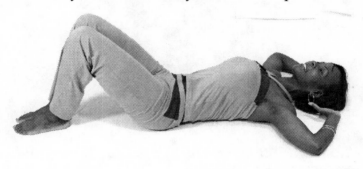

B. Lift your feet as you keep your knees bent forming a 90 degree angle between your thighs and torso

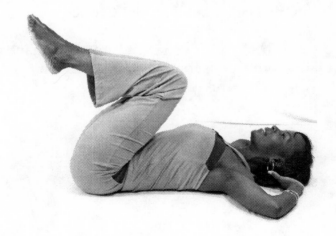

C. Simultaneously curl your pelvic bone toward your ribs and exhale as you lift your shoulders, bringing your knees toward your chest and your shoulder blades slightly off the mat.

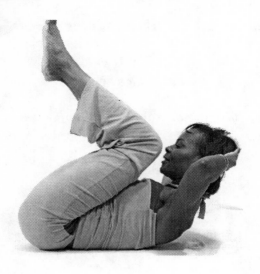

You should feel this in the upper and lower abdominal regions.
Release the contraction and try to complete 10-20 times, adding on as you become stronger

One Legged Abdominal Crunch #3

A. Lie on your back, relax your head into your hands, bend your left knee with feet flat on the floor and extend your right leg up, knee slightly bent

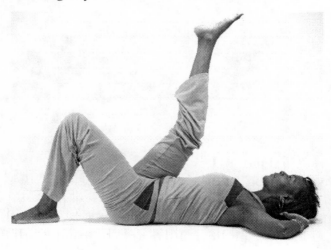

B. Lift your body up towards your right knee for 20 counts, focus on your chest going toward your knee, not your head

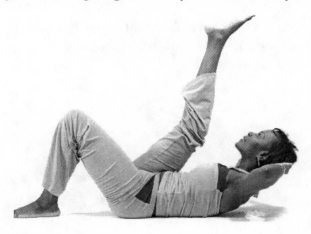

Keep your body lifted and switch legs, repeat on the other side

(Try to complete 20 on each side, adding on as you become stronger)

Rectus Abdominis Four Count Crunch   #4

A. Lie on your back, knees into your chest,
Hands behind your head, no pressure on the neck. Elbows even with the head and pointed out to the sides.

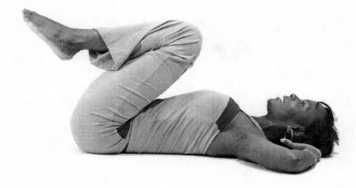

(If you're uncomfortable with your knees

into your chest keep your knees bent with
your feet flat on the floor).

B. Bring your upper body up towards your knees
in 2 counts. reach higher with hands forward
on # 3, and go back on #4

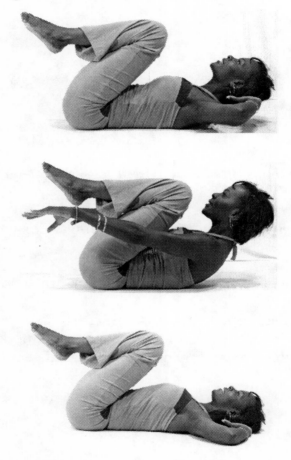

*Try to complete 10 sets. All 4 movements together equal one
set.*

The Hundreds (Rectus Abdominal) #5

It's very important to keep your upper body as high as possible. This helps reduce the strain on your neck, while strengthening your torso.

A. Lie on your back, knees are bent hands are underneath your thighs.

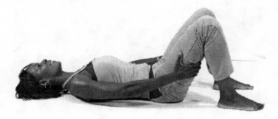

B. Lift the upper body as high as you can

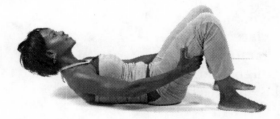

C. Hold position and raise hands above the head

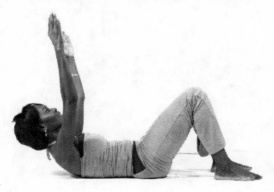

D. Keeping the upper body as high as you can bring your arms down until your palms are faced down about 2 inches from the floor)
Relax the upper body and press your hands down in a pulsing motion 20-30 times
Relax and try again

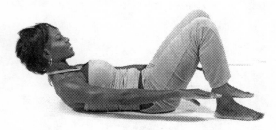

Rectus Abdominis Crunch (near a bed or chair) #6

A. Lie on the floor with your back flat and
knees bent, Place your lower legs
horizontally on top a bed or
Chair, Your thighs should be vertical,
your hips close to the chair or bed

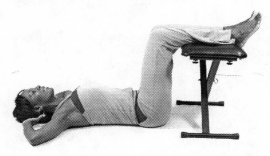

B. Curl up slowly with your upper back about
30 degrees off the floor, hold for 4 seconds,
relax, then repeat, try to complete 8-10 times
Adding on as you become stronger

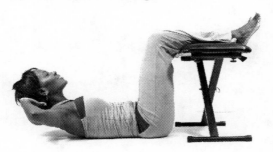

Advanced Rectus Abdominis #7

A. Sit on the floor with knees bent , hands on
your knees, back straight, shoulders down,
chest out and stomach held tight

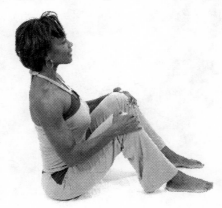

B. Lean backward, until your hands can
barely touch your knees
Hold movement for 16 counts (Do not hold
your breathe, Inhale and exhale as you're holding
the position

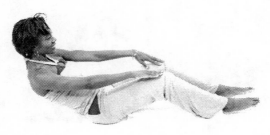

C. Keeping your hands on your knees pull
your body back up to a sitting position.

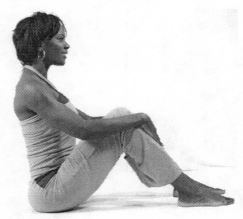

D. Stretch forward for 8 seconds, then repeat movement

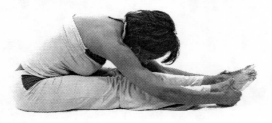

Try to repeat this exercise at least four times adding on as you become stronger. Remember if this exercise is too advanced, go to one of the previous stomach exercises until you become stronger.

Advanced Rectus Abdominis (Push-Up Position) #8

A. Place your body in a push up position. Arms Slightly bent, stomach tight, chest out, legs are Straight and your head is even with your back

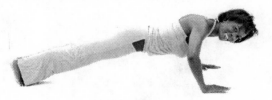

B. Bring your right leg in towards your chest as you slightly curl your back.

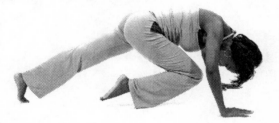

C. Uncurl your back, open up through the chest and extend that leg towards the back.

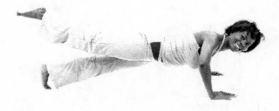

Repeat 5-10 times with the same leg before moving to the other side.

Advance Rectus Abdominis Exercise (Scissors) #9

A. Sit up on your elbows, with your upper body lifted, shoulders down and your chest is out, raise both legs in the air

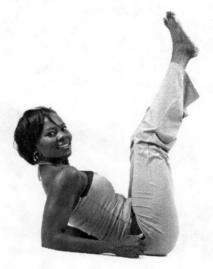

B. Bring your right leg down without touching the floor. Hold for 1-2 seconds, return to starting position. Continue by alternating the left leg without a break in between

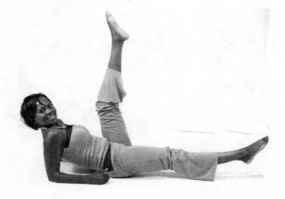

Try to complete 20 times, adding on as you become stronger

Again, remember your feet should never touch or hit the floor. If you're uncomfortable please wait until you're stronger and try again.

Advance Stomach Crunch Exercise with Extended Arms #10

A. Lie on your back with your legs straight and up in the air, Knees are slightly bent, keep the bottom of your feet Flexed and facing the ceiling

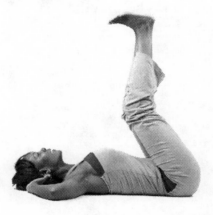

B. Lift your upper body off the floor with both arms reaching up towards your toes with a soft pulse for 8 counts

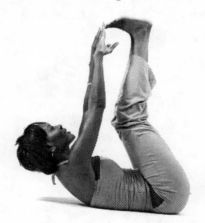

Relax for 4 counts and start again, trying to complete 8 different sets. Remember this is an advanced stomach exercise. If this position feels uncomfortable, go back to one of the previous crunches where you're supporting your neck until you become stronger.

Abdominal & Oblique Crunch #11

A. Lie on your back, legs up in the air, feet crossed at the ankle, knees are slightly bent, back is flat on the floor, hands behind the head, elbows Turned out to the side

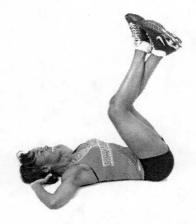

B. Lift your upper body off the floor, chin up towards the ceiling,

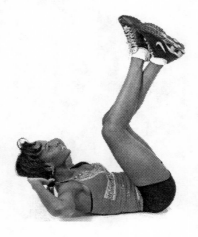

C. Move your upper body to the right, then middle, left, and then back to the middle never letting your upper body relax on the floor. (These 4 Moves together equal one set)

Try to complete 8 sets consecutively, adding on as you become stronger.

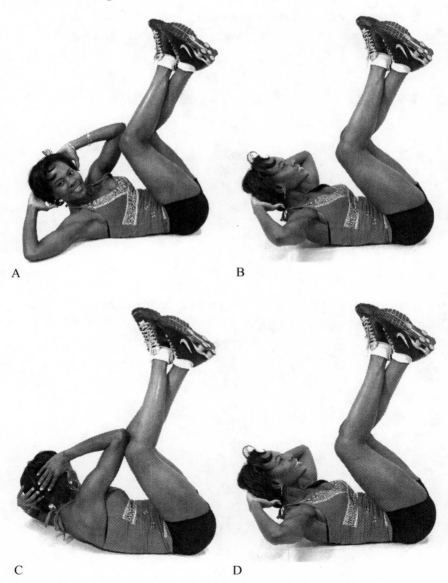

A   B

C   D

Are you uncomfortable on the floor? Try these stand up stomach exercises. They are great for everyone, but particularly designed for those with back problems and difficulty lying on the floor.

Stand Up Stomach Crunch #12

A. Standing with hands placed behind your head, (Try not to put unnecessary pressure on your neck)

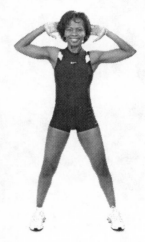

or you can place your hands in front of your chest.

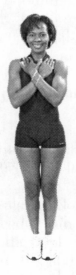

B. As you bring your upper body forward
Simultaneously raise your right knee then
    Your left knee towards your chest
without a break in between.

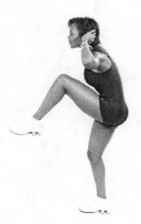

*Try to complete 20 repetitions, adding on as you become
stronger. Remember to continue contracting the stomach
muscles, keeping your head up as you inhale and exhale.*

Stand Up Stomach Crunch (turn thru the waistline) #13

A. Standing with knees slightly bent, stomach tight,
Shoulders down, chest out

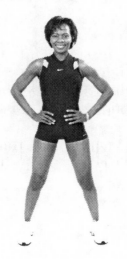

B. Bring your right arm across the front of your Body, pulsing for 8 counts

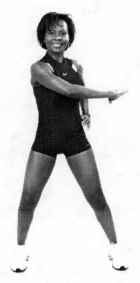

C. Repeat on the other side with your left arm across the front of your body, pulsing for 8 counts

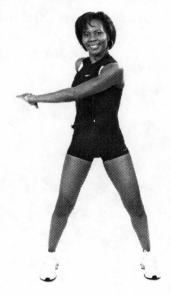

Try to complete eight sets of this exercise (each 8 count=1 set). When doing this exercise, keep your lower body stabilized, only focusing on moving your waistline, not your hips and thighs.

After exercising the stomach muscles you will need to stretch them afterwards. This stretch can keep those muscles loose and your belly flat.

Stomach Muscle Stretch (Foot Grab) #14

A. Stand near a chair or a wall for balance

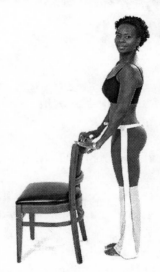

B. Bring your left foot backward toward your Left buttock until you can grab your ankle with your left hand, without arching your back, move your hips forward and keep your knees together

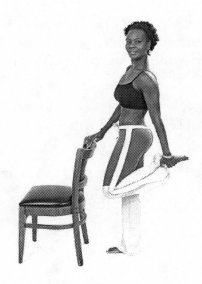

(Keep your stomach muscles tight and stay lifted)
Hold for 8 counts, repeat on the other side, try to complete a
total of 4 sets, 2 on each side

Standing Aerobic Trunk Twists

This is a good aerobic-type exercise that will help get your heart rate
up as well as burn calories throughout your waistline.

A. Stand with your feet shoulder width
apart and knees relaxed
Twist your torso to the left while keeping
your hips and legs as stable as possible.
As you twist to the left, cross your arm in
front of your body in a punching motion.

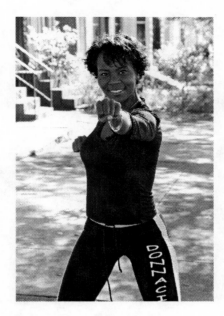

B. Twist back to the right and cross your left arm over your body in a punching motion.

Try to complete at least 100 repetitions without a break in between

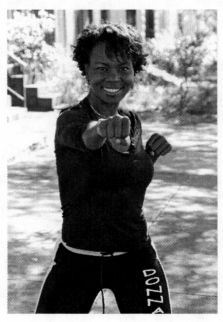

Walking Waistline Twist

Walking is considered one of the best forms of exercise because it's easy, convenient and inexpensive. So why not exercise your waistline at the same time. It doesn't require any special equipment and it can basically be done anyplace.

 Walk at a steady pace while swinging your arms through your waistline. Control your stomach
muscles and remember to stand as straight as you can. Your feet should step in a rolling action from the heel to the toe. Count to 100 before resting, then increase gradually.

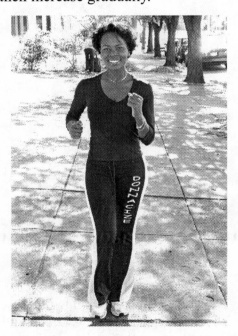

You can also walk with a furry friend for pleasure and safety, but the key is to exercise the waistline.

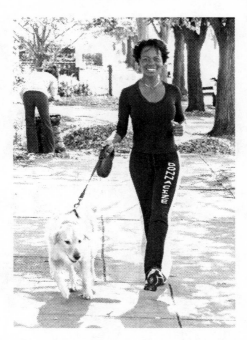

Control and Tighten Your Stomach Exercises
(While at Work)#15

I am very excited to introduce, stomach exercises you can perform at work. That's right, no fitness attire required and you don't need a babysitter or extra time. You can actually strengthen your stomach muscles while sitting at your desk. Try performing a couple of these exercises before lunch. This will not only shrink your stomach muscles, but it will help shrink your appetite as well.

While at work also remember that slouching forward accentuates your belly, but good posture is an instant belly flattener. So sit up straight, with your back flat and stomach tight. Bring your shoulders down and stick your chest out. Do not hold your breathe. Breathe normally.

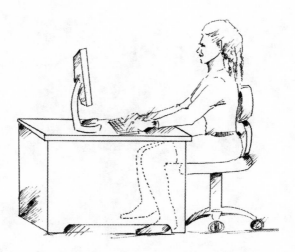

While sitting at your desk, contract your upper abdominal muscles by inhaling sharply and pulling in your abdominal area. Breathing normally, hold for 6 to 8 seconds, relax and repeat throughout the day.

Abdominal Crunch at Work   #16

A.   In a firm, armless chair, turn your body
away from the chair's back support.
Grab the chair's edges just in front of
your hips and hold the chair's back with your other hand.

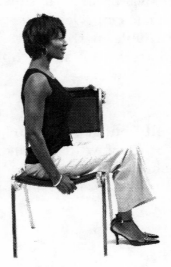

B. Exhale as you slowly draw your
knees up toward your chest
count #1

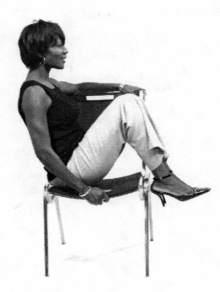

C. Inhale as you bring
your knees towards the front on #2

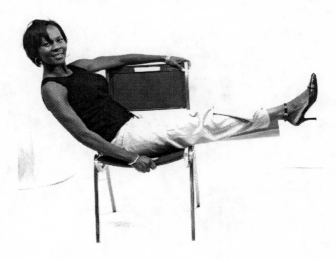

Hold onto the chair for balance and try to complete this exercise at least 10 times.

Stomach Curl (In a chair) #17

A. Sit in a chair and place your hands behind your head.

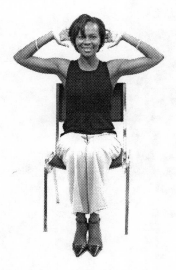

B. Move your head, neck and shoulders forward in one motion as you bring your right knee toward your chest.

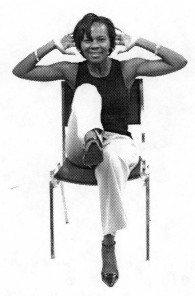

C. Return to starting position and repeat on the other side

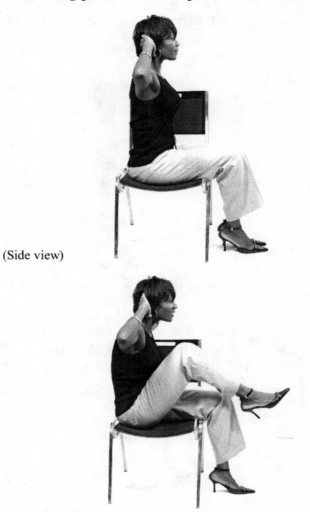

(Side view)

Be sure to contract your upper abdominal area as you crunch forward to meet your
raised knee. Come up on one and down on 2

Try to complete 5 on each side, adding on as you become
stronger

Abdominal Exercise at Work   #18

A. Sit up straight in a firm armless chair, feet are flat,
Your stomach muscles are tight, shoulders down
and your chest is out

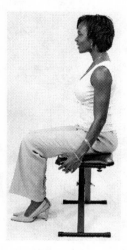

B. Take your right arm across the front of your
body with a soft easy pulse, twisting thru the
waist for 8 counts, repeat with your left arm

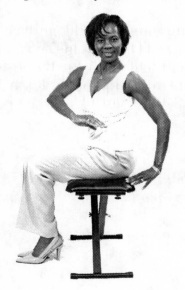

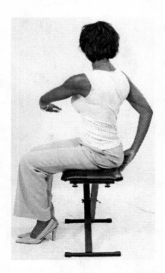

Remember to keep the hips and thighs centered, only moving thru the waist.
Try to complete 4 sets. 2 sets of 8 on your Right and two sets on your left side

Standing Abdominal Twist at Work #19

A. Standing, Legs shoulder width apart, hands are on your waistline, knees are slightly bent, stomach is tight, shoulders are down and your chest is out

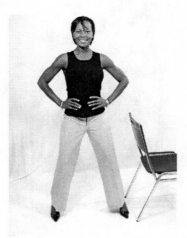

B. Twist towards your right for 8 counts

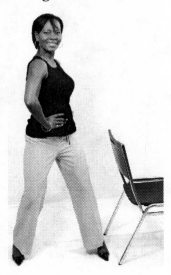

C. Twist towards your left for 8 counts

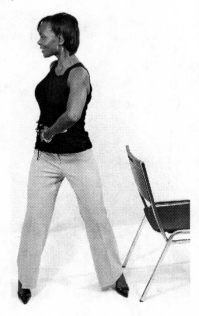

Try to complete 8 sets, four on your right and four on your left

Chapter 5:
Internal and External Oblique Exercises

The external oblique muscles originate at the side of the lower ribs and run diagonally to the rectus abdominis. These muscles wrap around your sides and are key to creating a wispy waistline. It is the external oblique muscles that provide definition in the side abdominal area and help to make your waist look smaller. The following exercises will help rid you of those love handles that you really don't love so much.

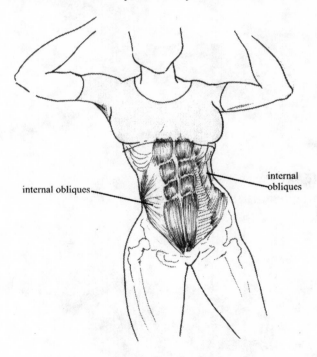

internal obliques

internal obliques

When performing oblique exercises, it is important not to pull on the neck to increase range of motion. During an oblique exercise, keep the abdominal area compressed and the legs and gluteal muscles relaxed with your chest open, aim your shoulder toward the opposite knee or hip versus the elbow.

The Basic Oblique Crunch #1

A. Lie on your back, place the outside of
Your right ankle on your left knee,
Turn your right knee outward,
Put your left hand behind your head with
your elbow pointed outward
Place your left arm on the floor
shoulder level, palm down

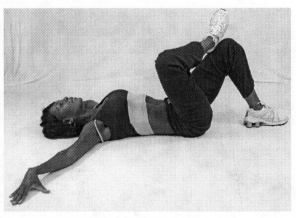

B. Slowly raise your left shoulder towards
your right knee, lifting your back
off the floor

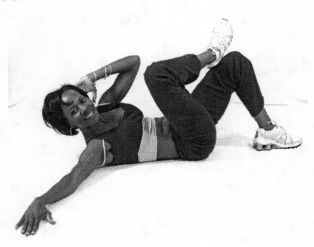

Complete 20 times slow and pulse 20 times fast before going to the other side, adding on as you become stronger.

Oblique Exercise (Stacked Knees) #2

A. Lie on your right side with your abdominal muscles contracted, ankles and hips are stacked and knees are bent
Place your left hand behind your head, and your right hand on your upper thigh

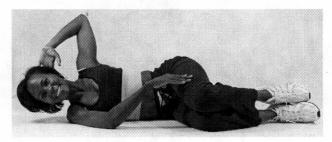

B. Lift your upper body off the floor so that your elbow points straight towards the ceiling (single count up and back)
Your thighs should not move, focus on your waistline

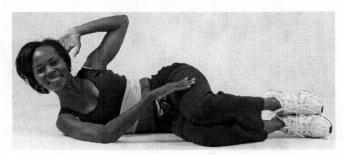

Try to repeat this exercise 20 times before moving to the other side. If you cannot complete 20 do as many as you can working up to 20. Turn your body to the left side and repeat.

Consult your physician if you experience back pain. If you have difficulty performing this stomach exercise, stick with oblique crunch number one until you become stronger.

Oblique Twist #3

A. Lie on your back
Bring your knees into your chest
Hands behind your head, elbows
pointed outward

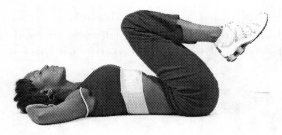

B. Alternate elbows from the right knee
to the left knee

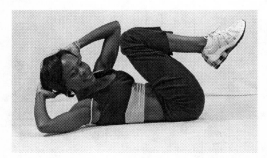

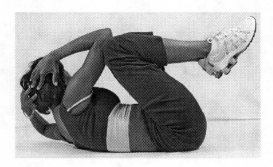

Try to complete 10 to 20 twist before adding on. Also remember to keep your back flat and your upper body in a relaxed position when performing the exercises.

Advanced Oblique Crunch #4

A. Lie on your back and bring your knees
into your chest
Hands are behind your head with your elbows
pointing outward

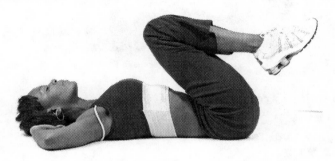

B. Take your right elbow to your left knee and
extend your right leg out towards the front as
low as you can without touching the floor

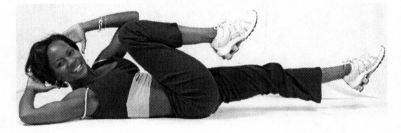

Repeat on the other side switching arms and legs

Repeat 2 sets of 20 resting in between sets. Remember to keep the back flat. If your back starts to arch, lift your leg higher until the back re-flattens. Lower your leg as you become stronger.

Advanced Oblique Crunch (Arms and knees to the side)
#5

A. Lie on your back, bring both knees into
your chest and lift your shoulders off the floor

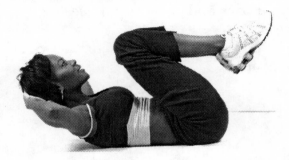

B. Reach both arms towards the outside of your
right knee, turn both knees to the left side,
pulsing for 8 counts

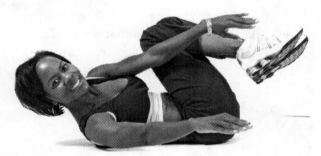

*Without a break between sets, repeat on the other side again
for 8 counts. Try to complete the right and left sequence three
times each before relaxing.*

Advanced Oblique Crunch (Stacked knees)   #6
*Unlike stacked knees #2, you are simultaneously lifting your
elbow and feet. If this is too difficult, stick with #2 until you
become stronger.*

A. Lie on your right side with your abdominal
muscles tight. Ankles and hips are stacked

and knees are bent
Place your left hand behind your head, and
your right hand on your upper thigh

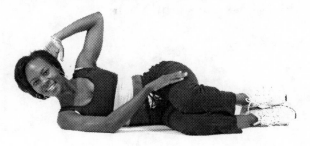

B.   Lift your upper body about 10 degrees off the
floor so that your elbow aim toward your
left hip as you lift your feet off the floor
(1 count up, and 1 count back)

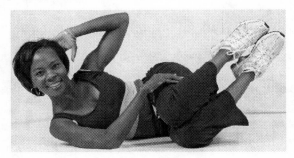

Keep your body steady and try not to rock back and forth.
Try to do 5 to 10 on each side, adding on as you become
stronger.

Standing Side Bends (Oblique Exercise) #7

A. Hands behind the head, elbows pointed out to the side, knees are slightly bent

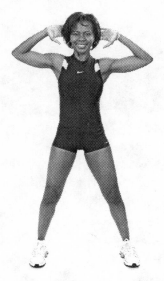

B. Lean to the right side with your elbows going towards your waistline for 8 counts

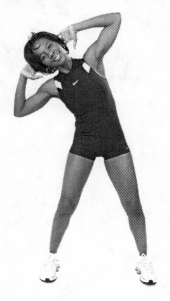

C. Repeat on the left side

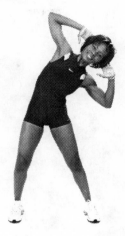

Try to complete 4 sets. Two sets of 8 on your right and 2 sets on your left

Standing Oblique Side Bends w/dumbbells #8

A. Legs are shoulder width apart, shoulders down, chest out, pelvic tilted. Knees are slightly bent. Hold a 3-5 pound dumbbells or two 16 ounce water bottles by your waistline.

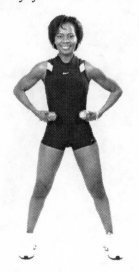

B. Put your Left hand on your waistline and your Right hand at your side. Lean towards your Right side, bending at the waistline.

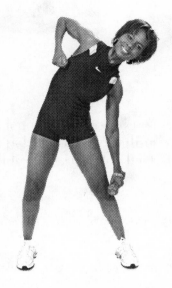

C. Lean towards your left side bending
at the waistline, 1 count down, 1 count up, repeat 10 times
return to neutral position and repeat on the other side

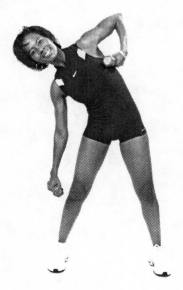

Repeat 10 times before going to the other side
Try to complete 4 sets of 10. Two sets of 10 on your Right and
two sets of 10 on your Left.

Standing Oblique Crunch (L-Position)   #9
With a Knee Lift

This exercise strengthens and defines your love handles. To
make this exercise more intense, you can add a 3 or 5 pound
dumbbell.

A. Stand with your feet about six inches apart,
put your right arm
in an L position with your palm facing the
front. Your left hand is on your waistline.

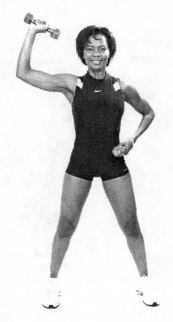

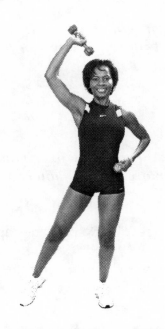

B. Bend at the waist while lowering your Right elbow and lifting your right knee. Squeeze your side abdominal muscle tightly. Repeat movement 10 times before going to the other side.

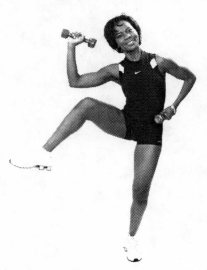

Exercise Your Oblique Muscles At Work
Seated Oblique knee lift #10

A. Sit in a chair with good posture, shoulders down, stomach tight, chest out, feet flat on the floor, hands behind the head

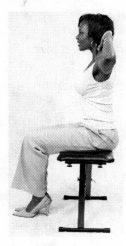

B. Take your right elbow towards your slightly raised left knee, up and down 8 times squeezing your abdominal muscles tight.

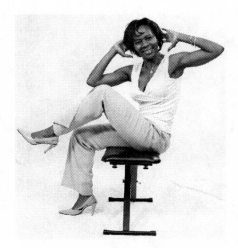

C. Repeat on the other side with your right hand on your waist and your left hand behind your head

Try to complete 4 sets, two sets of 8 on your right and left, adding on as you become stronger.

*Remember, when you are not accustomed to a particular exercise it can be uncomfortable. So always listen to your body. If you feel any pain, stop immediately and/or call your physician. If this exercise feels too difficult to complete, stay with the basic oblique crunches until you become stronger.

Oblique Twist (with a bar or dumbbells) #11

A. Sit in an armless chair, feet flat
on the floor Place a set of dumbbells or water
bottles on your shoulders.

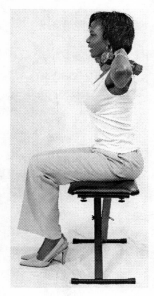

B. Twist to the Right and to the Left side

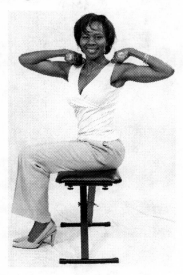

keep your stomach muscles tight and

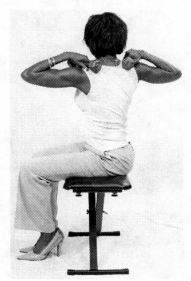

lower body stabilized.

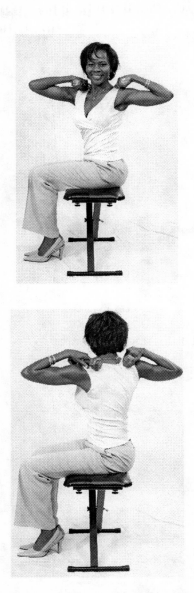

The dumbbells add resistance and force your body to work a little harder.

Standing Waistline Stretch #12

A. Knees are slightly bent, your stomach is tight,
Shoulders are down and your chest is out
Bring both arms up, clasping your hands
Together, palms facing the ceiling, stretch as high as you can.
(Hold for 8 counts)

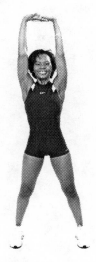

B. Keeping your hands together, stretch towards
Your right side and hold for 8 counts

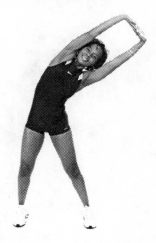

C. Back to the center

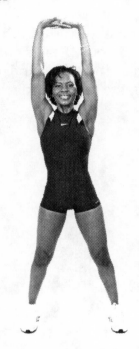

D. Repeat on the left side and stretch for 8 counts,

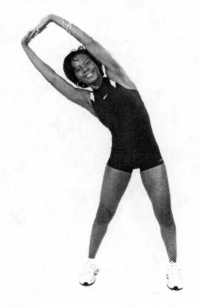

E. Come back to the center still
stretching keeping your palms towards the
ceiling and holding for 8 counts

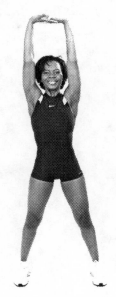

F. Curve your back bringing your arms in front
of your body, keeping your hands clasped
together (hold for 8 counts)

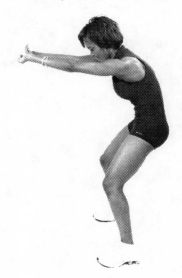

Bring your arms down and roll your body up. Repeat this entire stretch immediately after you complete your stomach exercises or whenever you feel tightness or soreness in your upper body, lower back or abdominal area.

Chapter VI
Lower Stomach Exercises

The entire rectus abdominous runs vertically from the chest bone (sternum) all the way down to the pelvic bone. Because the abdominal muscles are one big muscle group, you can't separate them, but you can target a specific area. The following exercises are designed to target the lower abdominal area.

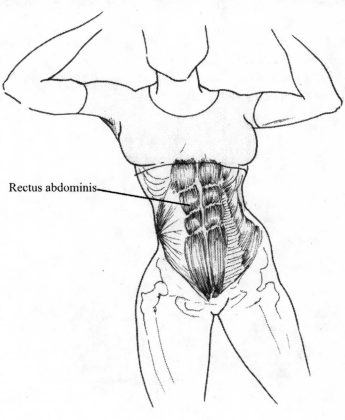

Rectus abdominis

Reverse Trunk Curl (legs in the air)   #1

The reverse trunk curl is one of the most beneficial abdominal exercises when attempting to restore lower abdominal muscles. This particular exercise puts more emphasis on the fibers in the lower part of the abdominal area because the contraction begins from the bottom of the muscle

Lift and lower your body without swinging. Try to do this movement at least 10 to 20 times adding on as you become stronger.

A. Lie on your back with legs in the air crossed at the ankle in a 90 degree angle, knees slightly bent, hands at your side, palms down

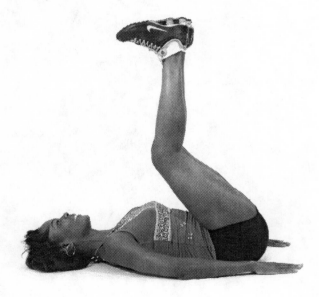

B. Slightly lift your buttocks off the floor and
Place your hands underneath your buttocks.
(This tilts the pelvic slightly up while supporting
the lower back)
This is your cushioning to prevent injury.
Your back and shoulder blades should
remain on the floor

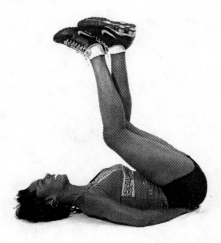

C. As you contract your abdominal muscles, curl your
pelvis upward, the bottom of your feet should face
the ceiling, your hips should rise only 3 to 5 inches
off the floor

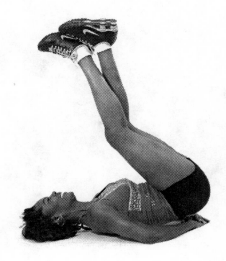

Maintain control throughout the movement and avoid rocking- or using momentum
Try to repeat at least 20 times, adding on as you become stronger

Lower Stomach (Curl in and Extend Out) #2

A. Lie on your back, with your head relaxed into your hands, elbows are pointed outward, chin up to the ceiling
Bring your knees into your chest

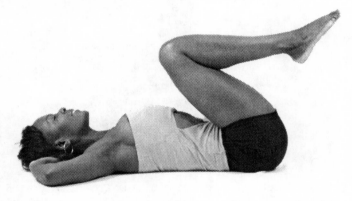

B. Lift your shoulders off the floor to meet your knees as they come in to your chest

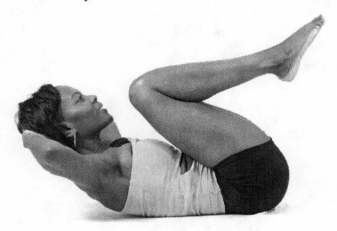

C. Lie back, extending your legs to the front as low as you can without arching your back and without your feet touching the floor

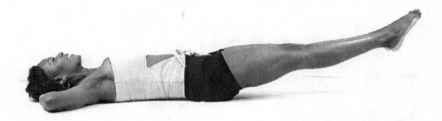

Repeat consecutively 10 to 20 times adding on as you become stronger.

Advanced Lower Stomach Curl In Extend Out #3

Follow steps A thru C in #2, the above exercise

D. Instead of lying back, keep your upper body lifted as you bring your legs in and extend them out. DO NOT lie back on the floor

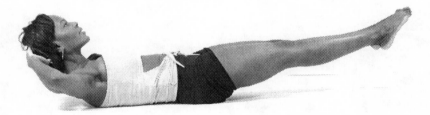

Push-Up Position (alternate knees)   #4

A. Body in a push up position

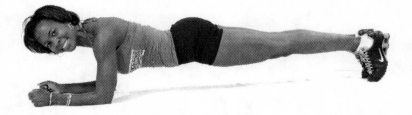

B. Bring your R knee down until it barely
touches the floor, bring it back up into the push
up position (Repeat on the left side)
Alternate right and left knee

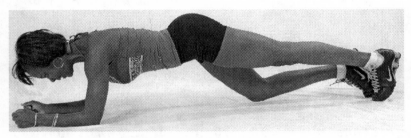

*Try to complete 10 times. Try to do 5 on the right and 5 on the
left. Relax and try again*
*Remember to keep your stomach muscles tight and your
body aligned (head, back, butt and legs in one line.*

Chapter VII:
You Can't Have A Small Waistline
Without A Strong Back

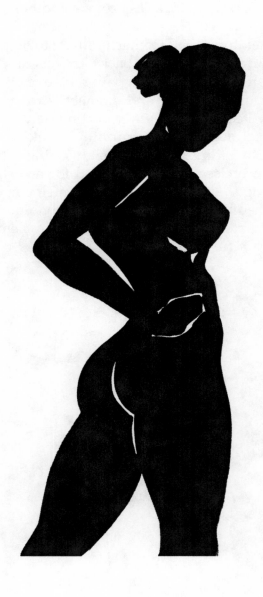

If I heard it once, I've heard it a thousand times, "I can't do certain exercises because I have lower back problems." No matter what our jobs, all of us use our back everyday when we're sitting, standing, lifting and even lying down. Many people suffer from back problems, due to a weakness in both their back muscles and abdominal area. When lifting weight, the abdominal muscles provide additional support for the spine as they contract and work together with the back muscles. Therefore, good stomach muscle tone is essential for correct posture and a healthy back. Exercising the back also minimizes problems with back pain with exercises that make the muscles in your back and stomach strong and flexible. Some people keep in good physical condition by being active in recreational activities like running, walking, biking and swimming. In addition to these conditioning activities, there are specific exercises that are directed toward strengthening and stretching the back muscles. So remember, not only are you strengthening your stomach with abdominal exercises, you are also ridding yourself of back problems now and gaining a beautiful waistline for the future.

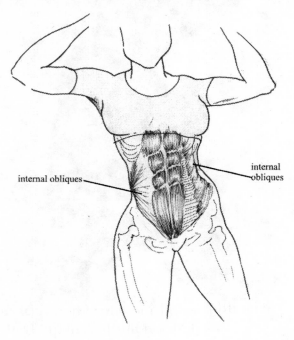

internal obliques

internal obliques

Back Exercise #1 (both knees to the side)

A. Lie on your back and pull both knees into
your chest

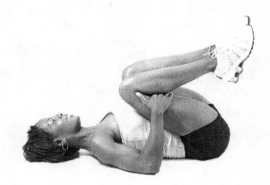

B. Turn both knees to your right side and turn
both arms to the left, hold for 10 seconds

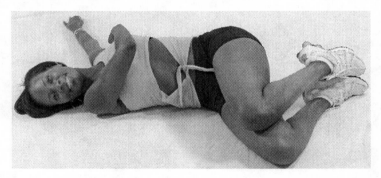

*Repeat on the other side, turning knees to your left and arms
to the right*

Back Exercise #2   (Superman lift)

A. Lie face down on the floor with legs
extended, toes are touching the floor
and arms are extended upward, palms down

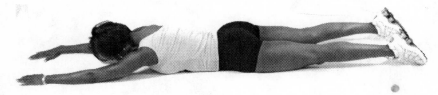

B. Keeping your head and neck aligned with
your spine, lift and hold
your right arm and left leg off the floor
for 4 counts

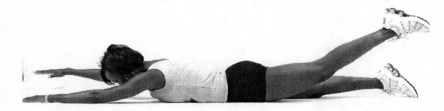

*Note- Keep your head down and repeat on the other side
alternating 4 on each side.*

Back Exercise (extended arms)   #3

A. Start by lying face down with your legs
Straight and toes tucked under

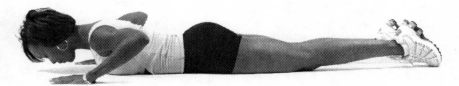

B. Bend your arms at your side, Palms flat
on the floor next to your chest,

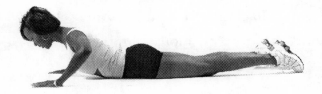

C. Lift your upper body up for 4 counts

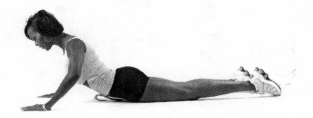

D. As your arms straighten, hold for 5-6

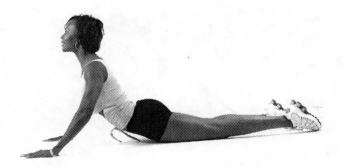

E. Relax on 7-8

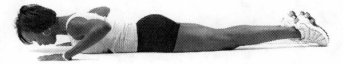

Repeat entire sequence at least 5 times
Come up on 1 thru 4, hold on 5-6, go back down on 7-8.

Back Exercise (table top)   #4

A. Body in a table top position. Hands and knees
on the floor, stomach muscles are tight.

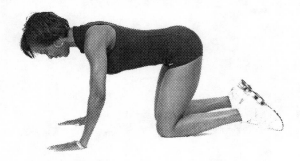

B. Keeping a flat back,
lift opposite arm and leg. Keep head
and leg aligned with the back.   Hold
for 4-8 counts .

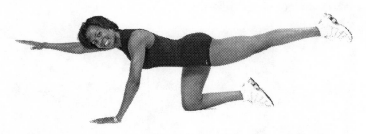

C. Repeat on the other side

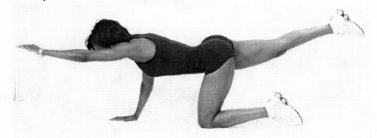

Try to complete 10 times, 5 on each side

Back Exercise (cat stretch hands and knees) #5

A. Body in a hydrant position, hands and knees on floor

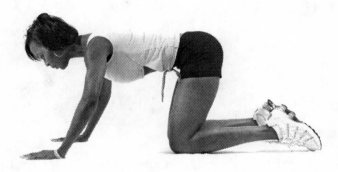

B. Keep the stomach muscles tight as you contract by putting a hump in your back, hold for 4 counts

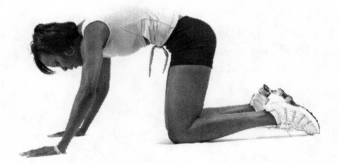

Flatten the back and try to complete this exercise at least five to ten times.

Relax the Back Cat Stretch   #6

A. Kneel on the floor with buttocks resting
on your heels , hands extended in front of
your body with head and neck resting
forward. Hold for 15 to 20 seconds

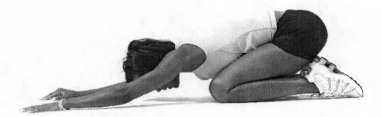

*You should feel this exercise in the upper, lower and middle
back areas.*

Advanced Lower Back Stretch #7

A. Lie on your back, knees are bent,
Hands grabbing the back of your thighs
just below the knee area

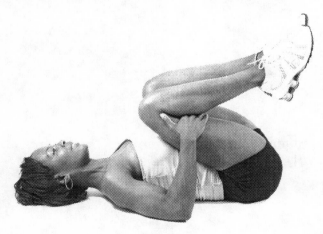

B. Gently pull your Right leg towards your
chest, while keeping your opposite
leg straight and as low to the floor as you possibly can.

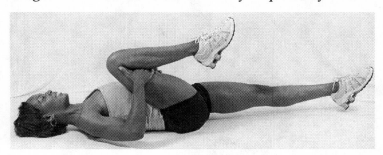

*If straightening your leg appears to be too difficult, keep
it slightly bent until your flexibility is enhanced. Repeat on
the other side holding for 8 counts each*

Stand-Up Back Stretch #8

A. Standing position: bend your knees and place
your hands on your thighs. Move your upper
body forward until your back is flat. Your
head, neck and back should be one even line

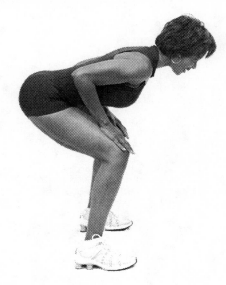

B. Contract your stomach muscles while arching
the back, keep your hands on your thighs,
and release by flattening the back at least
5 times.

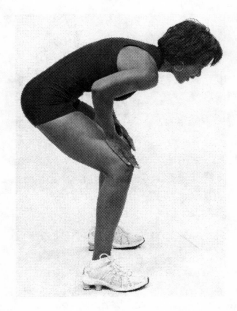

Section III:

Diet and Posture

Chapter VIII:
Healthy Meals and Snacks Made Easy

This chapter is designed to make your eating regimen a lot easier to implement. Included are great tips for dining out, breakfast, lunch, dinner, snack and recipe choices.

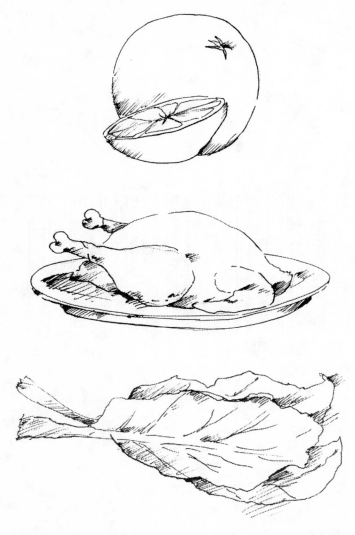

When you begin to change your diet and live a healthier lifestyle it's still okay to dine out once in a while, or on a regular basis, you just need to know the tricks of ordering. The following tips can help make dining in restaurants an enjoyable and healthy experience:

1. Before going to the restaurant, drink one or two glasses of water or eat a piece of fruit to curb your appetite.

2. Have a salad before the main course. Ask for salad dressing "on the side" and use it sparingly. You can also opt for a wedge of lemon or some seasoned vinegar instead of an oil-based dressing.

3. Avoid drinking wine or other alcoholic beverages before the meal. Alcohol stimulates the appetite and can also reduce your willpower.

4. When selecting a meal, avoid fried foods and try to choose dishes that don't include sauces, gravies or butter. It's okay to ask your server if your food can be prepared without high-fat ingredients or sauces. If you really want a taste of the sauce or gravy, ask for them "on the side."

5. If you decide to order dessert, choose fruit, sherbet or low fat vanilla ice-cream.

6. Dining companions can help by respecting your diet and not pressuring you into ordering rich dishes and desserts.

Dining out can be a very pleasant way to pass time with friends and family, and with a little effort can be easily integrated into an overall weight-loss program.

Breakfast

Most people fail to realize that breakfast is the most important meal of the day. It's your body's fuel that gives you more energy for the morning's task.   In addition, when you skip breakfast, you tend to eat larger lunches and dinners. The calories generated from these meals are much more difficult to burn since they are usually heavier and eaten later in the day when you are less active.

Below are healthy breakfast foods to make your choices a little easier:

Oatmeal: preferably the Quaker Old Fashioned, but the instant packages will do. To keep my oatmeal interesting I add fresh fruit (blueberries, apples, peaches bananas etc.) Each piece of fruit brings a new dimension to an old breakfast that I'm excited about all over again.

Wheat pancakes: are much healthier and less fattening than buttermilk pancakes/ Try topping them with a variety of fresh fruit, cool whip or low fat syrup

Bagels: whole grain, cinnamon and blueberry are very good without the cream cheese and butter.

Bran and high fiber cereals: ex. Raisin Bran, Wheaties and Special K

Soy, Rice or Skim Milk for pleasure or with cereal.

Fruit: apples, kiwi, bananas, mango, raspberries, strawberries, oranges and blueberries
It doesn't matter what your preference is, as long as you eat several pieces a day.

Egg whites also an excellent source of protein.

Nutrition Bars (at most supermarkets and health stores) A quick breakfast and a fast, simple and easy pick me up

Whole wheat or multi grain toast instead of white

A six egg omelette with vegetables (2 whole eggs and 4 egg whites) use your favorite vegetable.

English muffin toasted with light butter.

Try turkey bacon or chicken sausage instead of pork if you really want a meat for breakfast. Note- Some turkey or chicken sausage has just as much fat as pork, so be sure to read the nutritional label. Orange juice or green tea is healthier than coffee and can serve as a great substitute when you need that extra boost in the morning.

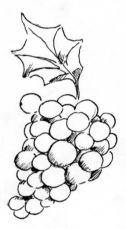

LUNCH

If you are not eating mini meals, lunch should be your heaviest meal of the day. A healthy filling lunch is crucial when concluding with smaller late evening meals. Try these lunch tips to assist you throughout the day:
* Eat healthy snacks in between meals to curb your appetite throughout the day.
* Substitute your white sandwich breads with wheat, rye or whole grain.
* Create a beautiful dark salad with sweet crunchy carrots, nice crispy cucumbers, dark lively broccoli, sweet juicy tomatoes

and tofu if you want the chewing sensation of meat without actually eating it.
* Use olive or canola oil when frying food.

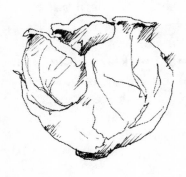

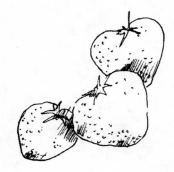

Need a few extra lunch ideas? Try these:

Sliced turkey or chicken breast on wheat or rye bread (adding lettuce and tomatoes to your sandwich fulfills some of your vegetable intake.

Tuna Fish: preferably albacore in spring water, you can eat it straight from the can or add a light mayonnaise

Cup of cooked or raw vegetables (eat as much as you like)

Cup of pasta with one teaspoon of olive oil

In the mood for a burger? Try a **turkey or tofu burger** instead of beef. They taste so good you may never go back to beef.

Fish, crab cake or shrimp sandwich

Bowl of soup with crackers
For a perfect pasta portion, keep a quarter piece near your spaghetti at home. It's diameter is exactly the size of the 2-ounce stac k(about 200 calories) that you should serve per person.

DINNER

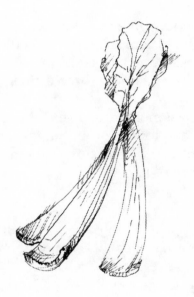

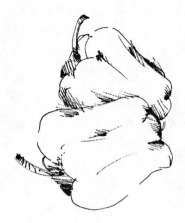

Many of the men and women I've spoken with say that dinner is the meal that gives them the most difficulty. What should I eat? What is the best time to eat? What shouldn't I eat? All of these questions bring us to the three dinner rules:

Rule #1: Eat your last meal three to four hours before bedtime. This period is needed for the proper digestion of food. This in turn prevents acid reflux, heart burn, stomach cramps and the unnecessary storing of fat.

Rule #2

Since dinner is your last meal of the day, you want it to be your healthiest meal for several reasons:
1. You're usually not as mobile. 2. Dinner time is usually wind down and relax with the family time so you don't want to feel bloated. And 3. This type of stillness does not allow your body to burn calories as rapidly.

Rule #3
Stay away from fried foods, heavy carbohydrates, juices, sodas and breads for your last meal of the day. These foods are extremely fattening and your body is too still to burn those calories.

Below are great dinner choices:

Fish baked or broiled- Seafood are an excellent source of protein and they're less fattening than other meats

A whole turkey or chicken- Be creative and make a healthy turkey soup one day and a turkey salad the next. Slice it up for sandwiches. You can even use the slices for your breakfast meat or on top your salad.

Meatloaf made with ground turkey instead of beef. (You'll feel much lighter after dinner. Also know that anything that you've used ground beef for in the past, can be substituted with ground turkey.

Baked or broiled potatoes. Not fried.

Brown rice instead of white

Spaghetti with ground turkey instead of beef

Vegetable or Meatless Lasagne

Any type/ assortment of vegetables (asparagus, string beans, collard, mustard or kale, etc.)

Baked or broiled skinless chicken

Beans any kind (very high in protein)

Sweet potatoes - baked whole, boiled or sliced with light seasoning. You can even cut them like french fries and bake them in the oven or fry them in olive oil.

Grilled Eggplant

Vegetable or chicken stew

Homemade chicken soup with plenty of vegetables

I came across these recipes that sounded exciting yet simple so I had to try them. These recipes came out great even for me. Please try them.

Baked Chicken and Noodles
1 medium-size chicken, cut into 8 pieces, skin removed
1 teaspoon poultry seasoning
1/4 teaspoon ground black pepper

1/8 teaspoon salt (optional)
1 small onion, chopped small
1 small green bell pepper, sliced thin
2 cans low- or no-fat cream- of-chicken soup
4 cups dry wide no-egg-yolk noodles
Optional garnish: chopped parsley
Heat oven to 400 degrees, lightly coat large baking dish or small roaster pan with cooking spray. Place chicken pieces in dish; sprinkle with seasonings. Top chicken with onion and bell pepper. Pour soup over chicken, add 2 soup-cans water to pan. Bake one hour. Meanwhile cook noodles according to package directions. Stir noodles into dish with chicken on top. Bake 25 additional minutes. Sprinkle with parsley and serve. Makes 6 servings.
Per serving: 476 calories, 33 grams protein, 8 grams fat, 65 grams carbohydrate, 787 milligrams sodium, 68 milligrams cholesterol.

Vegetable Soup To Die For

7 cups canned low-sodium vegetable or chicken broth
1 medium-size leek, white and light-green parts only: halved lengthwise, cut into 1-inch lengths, washed throughly.
1 celery rib, sliced
6 small red potatoes, un peeled, cut into 1-inch chunks
½ small head cabbage, cored, shredded or chopped
16 - ounce can stewed tomatoes
2 medium -size carrots sliced
2 tablespoons chopped fresh parsley or tarrogan
1 teaspoon salt (optional)
½/ teaspoon ground black pepper

In large saucepan over medium heal, bring broth to simmer. Add leek, celery, potatoes, cabbage, tomatoes and carrots. Simmer until potatoes are tender, about 10 minutes. Stir in parsley. Season with salt (if desired) and pepper. Ladle into bowls and serve immediately. Makes about 6 servings. Personalize this recipe by adding your favorite vegetables or leftovers   From the refrigerator. Just stir them into the mix and simmer.

Per serving: 129 calories, 6 grams protein, 1 gram fat, 27 milligrams carbohydrate, 636 milligrams sodium, 0 milligrams cholesterol

Shrimp Fried Rice

What a delicious way to use leftover rice. Or plan ahead and cook the rice in advance and refrigerate it so the grains will separate and not become mushy when stir-fried.

1/4 cup low sodium soy sauce
½ teaspoon sugar
1/8 teaspoon ground black pepper
1/8 teaspoon cayenne pepper
2 tablespoons peanut oil or vegetable oil.
3 cups cooked small or medium- size shrimp
1 cup fresh bean sprouts, rinsed, drained
1 cup cooked green peas or frozen mixed oriental vegetables
1 scallion, sliced thin
2 large eggs, lightly beaten
½ of 7 ounce jar roasted red peppers, diced
optional garnishes: lemon wedges, chopped or whole scallions
In small bowl, blend soy sauce, sugar and black and cayenne peppers; set aside. In large 12- inch nonstick skillet or wok, heat oil over medium heat. Rotate skillet until oil covers bottom. Add rice; cook, stirring quickly and pressing out any lumps, about 5 minutes. Add shrimp, bean sprouts, green peas and scallion; stir-fry 2 minutes. Move rice mixture to side of skillet, add eggs. Cook, stirring constantly, until eggs are cooked through but still moist. Stir eggs and roasted red peppers into rice mixture. Next stir in soy-sauce mixture; cook until heated through, about i minute. Garnish as desired. Serve hot. Makes about 4 servings.

Per Serving: 351 calories, 19 grams protein, 10 grams fat, 45 grams carbohydrate, 765 milligrams sodium, 189 milligrams cholesterol

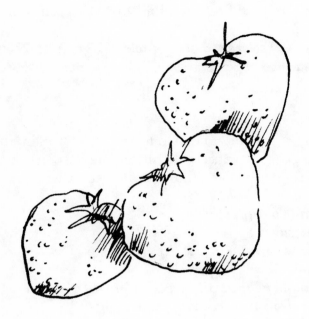

Strawberry-Blueberry Trifle

For a bit of added indulgence, serve with scoop of fat-free frozen vanilla yogurt. Make about 6 servings.

Serving size 1 to 10

1 Entennman Fat Free Golden Loaf
1 cup sliced fresh strawberries (cup size will vary depending on serving size)
1 cup cool whip

Cube cake into bike sized pieces. Line bottom of trifle or dish with cake cubes. Layer with cool whip. Cover with strawberries and blueberries. Repeat steps again starting with cake cubes. Delicious and easy.

Per serving: 160 calories 0 fat, o cholesterol

It's Snack Time

Few of us can resist the temptation of sweet food. Sweets go hand in hand with parties, celebrations, and rewards for good behavior. One way to curb a sweet tooth is to find nutritious alternatives to high-calorie desserts. Whether you're at the mall, in the car, or at work, keep yourself armed with healthy snacks to help you resist fat-and-calorie-laden temptations from vending machines and fast-food stores. If you're going to snack, limit it to two per day in-between mealtimes. Below are some healthy options to make your snacking more enjoyable and low-fattening.

A nutrition bar - try something close to a balance bar. My favorite is chocolate coated and Nature Grains Oatmeal Raisin by GeniSoy™ - each bar supplies 14 grams of soy protein

Fruit- bananas, mango, strawberries, apples, oranges, kiwi, raspberries, pears, etc.

Quaker fruit and oatmeal bars - (strawberry cheesecake is delicious)

A cup of instant bean soup - fiber packed and filling, just add water

Grape Nuts Cereal with dried cranberries or raisins

Yam Potatoes - this is more than a side dish, it's actually a great snack

If you crave ice-cream try **Haagen Dazs Low Fat Vanilla Ice-Cream,** it's 200 calories less than regular ice-cream and only 19 grams of saturated fat per cup

Entenmann's Fat-Free Raspberry Danish has a buttery crust, a wonderful sweet filling and it's 80 calories less than a regular Danish

Lions and tigers and bears: oh my- **animal crackers** are only 12 calories each

Low-fat string cheese (2 oz) The perking power of protein and the rich taste of cheese without all that nasty fat

Ryekrisp or wheat crackers

Nuts- pistachios, almonds, cashews or shelled

Cucumbers - try slicing and eating them alone or with a little vinegar and water

Baby carrots are very sweet and crunchy

Dried fruit like prunes, apricots, bananas, raisins or cranberries

No-oil baked tortilla chips

Popcorn (air-popped or "light")

Raw vegetables with nonfat or low fat dip

Unsweetened ready-to-eat cereals

Fresh or Frozen Grapes

Eat a frozen fruit bar instead of a popsicle

Use vanilla yogurt instead of oil in brownie recipes to cut down on fat

The snacks you choose also play a big part in keeping you healthy, so keep low fat snacks on hand to curb that appetite throughout the day.

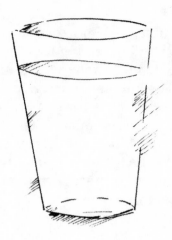

WHY DRINK WATER??????

I always consider myself a work in progress. So when I say I use to drink one glass of water per day, believe it. Now I drink 6 to 8 glasses daily. You too can increase your water intake. Water makes up half our adult body weight and provides a medium for all of the body's fluids which are vital for breathing, digestion and metabolism. The only thing more important than water for our body is the consumption of air. Water balances the acids in the body and carries nutrients into all the body's cells and is essential for removing waste from cells. When you don't drink enough water, problems such as dehydration, sore muscles, joints and digestive inefficiency can occur. It doesn't matter whether you are dieting or not, you should drink at least eight 8 ounce glasses of water per day. If drinking this much water is difficult in the beginning, start with four glasses and try diluting your juices and non-caffeinated fluids.

Remember, coffee, black teas and many soft drinks contain caffeine. If you thirst for something besides plain water, try herb teas, caffeine free soft drinks or juice.

Donna Lynn

The human brain sends off signals telling us when we are hungry or thirsty. Unfortunately, these signals are simultaneous so we end up eating food when the body's only desire is thirst. Remember, don't wait until you are thirsty to drink water, that is usually the first sign of dehydration. Many of my clients say their reason for not drinking much water is simply because it's not pleasurable. I tell them not to focus on the taste, but the benefits instead. Water cleans the body as it assists in purging toxins to help organs function better. If you are still not convinced here are a few additional reasons to support your increase of water:

1. Water helps you to eat less. Next time you feel hungry, curb your appetite with a glass of water.
2. Everyone loves glowing skin. Same comparison, water in, healthy skin out.

Also, realize that almost all foods contain water, with the largest amount being found in fruits. To help your water intake, try carrying a bottle of water with you throughout the day. You will be amazed by your consumption. Last but not least, try drinking a glass of water first thing in the morning, this will get you off to a healthy start.

One final note: When you first increase your water intake to the recommended level, you will probably need to urinate more frequently. Your bladder will adjust after a few weeks, and you'll urinate less frequently but in larger amounts.

112

Chapter IX:
Good Posture... Why Is It So Important?

When talking about good health, good posture is as important as eating right and exercising. Why? Because without good posture, it is extremely difficult to be physically fit. The appearance of a physically fit body can look unfit and sluggish in seconds with poor posture, believe me, I know. When stressing the importance of posture with my clients, I have this habit of using myself as the model. They are always shocked and amazed at the transformation from looking fit and strong, to unfit. As embarrassing as it is for me to demonstrate (because I want to look fit at all times), I realize that it's a major lesson in posture that won't be forgotten.

WHAT DOES GOOD POSTURE MEAN?

Good posture simply means that your bones are properly aligned and your muscles, joints and ligaments can work as nature intended. It also means that your vital organs are in the right position and can function at peak efficiency. It doesn't matter what age you are, how you carry yourself when working, relaxing or playing can have big effects. I've included a posture self test that you can perform at home. In order to perform this self-test you must be able to see the lines and curves of your body, so please wear fitted attire, or nothing at all.

THE MIRROR SELF-TEST FOR POSTURE PROBLEMS

Front View - Stand facing a full length mirror and check to see if:

1. Your shoulders are level

2. Your head is straight

3. The spaces between your arms and sides seem equal

4. Your hips are level and your knee caps are straight ahead

5. Your ankles are straight

If you find minimal imbalances within your posture, you may want to start paying more attention to these areas that appear to be off balance.

For example, if your shoulders are not leveled, you may have a habit of carrying an oversized bag or heavy pocket book consistently on the same shoulder. This is probably the most popular mistake men and women unconsciously make in creating bad posture. This was actually my first experience with bad posture. As an aspiring dancer and fitness enthusiast I constantly put tennis shoes, dance attire, water bottles and anything else I felt necessary into my bag. One day I looked into the mirror and there I was, leaning toward my right side. This postural problem was corrected by first carrying a lighter load and secondly, switching my bag from my right to my left side. This led me to consciously pay more attention to shifting my weight evenly.

If you find major imbalances within any of the areas we spoke of in the mirror test, try to pay special attention to these areas. If that doesn't help, you may need professional help to restore the normal curves of your spine.

HOW DO YOU KNOW IF YOU HAVE GOOD POSTURE?

Good standing posture is when the following are properly aligned:

From the front, your shoulders, hips and knees are of equal height

From the side, you can easily see the three natural curves in your back

Your head is held straight, not tilted or turned to the side

From the back, the little bumps on your spine should be in a straight line down the center of your back.

Obviously, no one spends all day in this position, but if you naturally assume a relaxed standing position, you will carry yourself in a more balanced position and with less stress in your other activities.

FINAL POSTURE NOTE OF ENCOURAGEMENT

Good posture will have you looking years younger. Poor Posture will make you look older than you are. When you are slumped over, or hunched over, not standing straight, you can add years to your appearance. For women, the more rounded the shoulders, the more stomach and breasts may sag. It doesn't matter what age a woman is, any woman can help reduce the sag in her belly and her breasts by nearly 50% by simply standing tall.

Section IV

Commitment

&

Motivation

Chapter X:
Questions I Am Most Often Asked

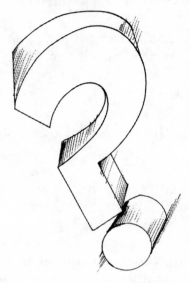

The following are several questions I'm often asked:

How long will it take to lose my stomach?

I am always extremely honest with my clients when I tell them "Don't expect to lose your stomach overnight." Although its important to practice patience, I also promise that they will see a difference within a four week period if they exercise cardiovascularly 3-4 times per week and complete their abdominal, back and oblique exercises. This with a healthy diet and good posture is the lifetime formula for success. As I said earlier, the reality is that you must commit, and it will take some time, but the rewards will be plentiful.

Can I still perform the stomach exercises with lower back pain?

You should first consult with your physician and schedule an exam. This way you have an idea of why you're having the back pain and what exercises you can perform without further damage to that area.

When is the best time of day to exercise?

Whenever you have the time to exercise is always the best time. Whether it's early morning or late evening, just do it. I'm sometimes asked if the body burns more calories in the morning than it does in the evening. The short answer is: It doesn't matter. Some people are full of energy and life early in the morning, while others need more time to be motivated. Work with what is right for you. As long as you're moving, you can never go wrong.

I feel fine, so why should I exercise?

There are lots of good reasons for exercising. Exercising heightens the functions of your body. Your heart and lungs work at a higher capacity when you're fit. Regular exercise also plays an important role in weight control. Even if you're not overweight, a strong, healthy, fit body is still beneficial to function at a higher level at work and at play. Still not convinced, keep reading:

...exercise can prevent disease and premature death
...can improve the overall quality of your life
...helps relieve emotional and nervous tension
...can have you feeling 10 years younger
...you look and feel better

Should I Eat, Before or After I Exercise

If you decide to eat before exercising, be sure to give the body at least ninety minutes for food digestion before physical activity and two to three hours for a very large meal. Your body works extra hard if it's trying to break down food intake and send extra blood to your working muscles all at once.

Should I Exercise If I'm Feeling Soreness?

After starting an exercise program, muscle soreness is quite normal for the first few weeks. This is the result of slight internal swelling in the fibers of the ligaments and tendons connecting the muscles. If you feel sore the next day, smile and know that those previous sleeping muscles are now awake.
*Important Note - If you feel **major** discomfort and pain, stop exercising and consult your physician.

Is It Okay To Take A Break From Exercising?

While it's important to exercise regularly to see physical gains, don't feel you can't take a day or two off. You need time to adapt to the physiological changes occurring in your body. Muscles generally take 48 hours to repair and rebuild. Rest also aids in the removal of metabolic waste products, such as lactic acid (the chemical responsible for muscle soreness and fatigue). You need rest to perform your best.

Chapter XI:
Feeling Good About You

Feeling Good About You _

One sure way to feel good about your outer beauty is to start with your inner beauty. You are embarking on a major lifestyle change that will enhance the way you look, feel, eat, drink, and yes, dress. Doing great things for your body like eating healthy foods, drinking water and exercising will lead to a higher energy level and a lower stress level. I really want you to remember that reshaping your body does not and will not happen overnight. So be patient and enjoy the positive ride. Now the best thing about this ride is that it is achievable with your goals being the destination.

Below are steps to help keep you on track with the three goals you made earlier.

1. **Stay focused** - Always remember why you picked up this book in the first place and let that continue to be your motivation.

2. **Stick with your plan** - That specific day and time you chose earlier is your 15, 30 or 45 minute take care of me time. Remember, there is nothing wrong with being a little selfish.

3. **Have fun**- This is not meant to be a grueling experience. Taking care of yourself could and should be fun.

4. **Keep it interesting** - change your aerobic activity as often as you like. You can invite family and friends to join you, but don't depend on them. Remember your goal is to lose **YOUR** stomach _

Chapter XII
<u>You Are Not Alone</u>

I absolutely love watching lives evolve for the better. When you become healthier your entire mental and physical state is automatically enhanced. When I receive letters and phone calls from people whose lives have been changed, I too am also changed. People want to share their weight loss stories and battles with me. I appreciate this and do not take them or their situation lightly. The progress reports in this chapter are meant to shed light on a variety of issues and concerns. Whether it's the yo, yo diets, the lack of energy, difficulties focusing on a healthy lifestyle or the unhappiness felt when alone. Many men and women will see themselves within some element of these letters. Exercising regularly is one of the most positive habits you can develop. Not only will it change your life, but your new lifestyle will effect your children, friends co-workers and family members. You owe it to yourself to live the most energized and fulfilling life that you possibly can. Please read on and be inspired and most importantly remember, **<u>YOU ARE NOT ALONE.</u>**

MELANIE'S STORY

Hello, My name is Melanie and I_use to be addicted to diets. It didn't matter if it was a cabbage diet, pills, capsules, all carbs, liquid or slim fast diet, everything was a possibility for me to lose my nine month baby stomach, that was missing the baby. Now I am 30 pounds lighter with an additional 6 inches off my waistline. Yes, 6 inches. I met Donna at a health convention. I found her to be very personable, knowledgeable and approachable. Afterwards I patiently waited to speak with her. Donna took time to guide me through the steps needed to lose my weight. Since I lived too far to attend her classes, she gave me a video tape and we agreed on a workout schedule that we shook and hugged on. We converse by e'mail at least twice per week.

Now eight months later I am still exercising the Donnacize Way. Now I can chase the bus that I want to get on and catch it. You only need determination to Donnacize. Excuses weigh more than the person making them. Believe me, I know. You have everything to gain and nothing to lose so be determined and stick it out. You owe it to yourself to be the best you can be. Believe me, if I can do it, you definitely can.

TANYA'S STORY

I am writing this letter as I return from Atlanta, GA. This is my first working trip since I've been Donnacizing regularly for three months. Even though I have been away for five days, I did not fail to spend at least 30 minutes each day exercising. Additionally I made choices to walk, or take the steps instead of the elevator. Before bedtime after my teeth were brushed it was time to exercise my stomach muscles. I absolutely must brush my teeth before bed so I made a personal rule that if my teeth were brushed before bed, my stomach muscles will also be tightened before bedtime. This may not seem important to some, but for me it reflects a new mind set. A year ago it would not have occurred to me to get up at 6:00am to ride a bicycle. I still wanted a smaller waistline, but to work for it was unthinkable. So how did this change occur? The answer is simple...... Donnacize

I met Donna thru a friend who absolutely loved exercising with her. I found Donna to be genuine and committed to each individual. She actually knew the entire class by name. If you doubt yourself, then join the club. If you think it's impossible to change your body, then join the club. If you hate the sight of your body, then again, join the club. You are not alone, all of us have feelings of doubt. But when you start to do something about it, your confidence is heightened and your doubt subsides. To be perfectly honest, the first couple of classes nearly killed me, but I kept going back. I was broken down and sore, but I was happy. If you're just starting the Donnacize program, don't get discouraged. Just stay true to your commitment to yourself and the rewards will be plentiful.

MICHAEL'S STORY

It's been over a year since my fiance' introduced me to Donna. He would come home telling me how much he enjoyed exercising at Donnacize. I found my fiance' full of energy, less stressed and most importantly, we saw physical change.

Now he is concerned about his own health and I no longer make his doctor appointments. He does it himself, "regularly". He has become a much healthier eater, and he exercises five days per week. He suggested that I stop by one day to meet donna and see for myself. I took one trip and I also became a member. Donna will whip you into shape and have you feeling good about yourself. You create your own goals and strive to reach those goals at your own pace. There is no pressure, stress, or competition with anyone other than you.

We now speed walk and hike together on weekends. Our new lifestyle is filled with energy, passion and an eagerness to exercise. If you feel uncomfortable at the large fitness centers (like we did) there are many other things you can do to get in shape. My fiancé walks 10 blocks one direction and back when he is not exercising with Donna. Once you incorporate fitness into your lifestyle there is no turning back. Donna helped change our lives for the better, and I can promise that she can do the same for you.

Patricia's Story/ Doing It The Right Way

Hi, my name is Patricia and I am 100 pounds lighter that I was two and a half years ago. How did I do it? Starting at the weight of 310 pounds did not make it an easy task. I was tired and angry most of the time and even though I worked two jobs, I was very inactive. It was so bad that I could not walk to and from my car without being exhausted. What was even sadder was the fact that I could not keep up with my children. In 2003, I reached my turning point after viewing myself on a home video. I could not believe it! I never really looked at me.

Well, there I was, all 310 pounds of me. I prayed, I cried, and then I went into action. In the course of my lifetime battle with weight loss, I have tried everything from diet pills to Jenny Craig. They all work or don't work to a certain degree. Always remember, no diets work unless you work it. With the help of my exercise program and nutritionist, I learned a new way of eating and exercising. My progress was steady. During the course of the next year and a half, I loss a total of 110 pounds! No I am not a size 8, and I still have 40 more pounds to lose. I wish I could tell you that there is a short cut or magic cure, but there isn't. Losing weight the right way through proper diet and exercise is the only way, and yes, it is hard work.

Once I reached the next level I needed another challenge and that was Donnacize! After just one class, I knew I was home. I was whipped, but I was happy. The more I exercised, the stronger I became. The atmosphere at Donnacize is overwhelming. We are like family. Donna's personality shines most, and it is that personality that has drawn so many to her. At Donnacize I learned to challenge myself, and to reach for new goals. Emphasis is placed on health, fitness and lifestyle change. Today, thanks to Donna and healthy eating, I've been able to keep my weight off for the last two years. I can do up to two one hour aerobic classes if I choose to. I was able to complete a five mile walk or jog-a-thon, and needless to say, I can get to and from my car very easily. The best part is not only can I keep up with my children, I can keep up with my grandchildren! I also have returned back to school. I am completing my second year in college, ultimately receiving my degree as a Registered Nurse. Life for me now is all brand new. I thank God and I thank his angel Donna!

SARA'S STORY

Hello, My name is Sara, and I have lost over 50 pounds since late November 2003 with Donna Lynn. I started Donnacizing after a friend constantly talked about her. When I complete my eight hours on the job I head straight home and exercise with my Donnacize Video. You see, just as my job is a necessity, so is my health. You have got to do this for you! I have tried fad diets without exercise, only to become twice as fat once I've depleted the pills or they no longer worked. In fact, I could have started my own pharmacy. The days when I watched my sizes creep up, while my stamina continued to go down are also gone. I do not fall asleep as soon as I get home. I do not eat as much. I have found confidence within myself and lowered my stress factors. I am more vibrant, limber and three times stronger. I use to hate my lower stomach with a passion. If I had a dollar for every time someone asked, "When is the baby due"? I could have retired from work. Those days are also gone. Lower stomach exercises only work when you do the cardiovascular exercises with them. Although it is difficult for me to attend Donnacize classes, I call her at least once per week. At first I kept asking, Donna when will I see a difference? When? When? When? Donna kept telling me to be patient, it will come. As discouraged as I was at times, I kept pushing forward in spite of it all. Then one day I slipped into a pair of jeans that I usually struggle to get into. There I was, shocked and smiling at the same time. My advice to you is to work hard and be patient, then one day you too will look into the mirror and say, "Yes, it's working, and I'm worth it"!

At this time I would like to thank you for choosing my book. I wish you all the success in the world with your new healthy lifestyle. Just remember.... if you really want it, You can have it. Please visit me on the web at www.donnacize.com or contact me at donna@donnacize.com.. I would love to hear from you.